Fabulously Fertile

Supercharge your fertility naturally

Sarah Clark CPC

Fabulously Fertile: Supercharge your fertility naturally

ISBN: 1500977616
ISBN 13: 9781500977610
Library of Congress Control Number: 2014915464
CreateSpace Independent Publishing Platform
North Charleston, South Carolina

The content of this book is for general instruction only. Each person's
physical, emotional and spiritual condition is unique. The instruction
in this book is not intended to replace or interrupt the reader's relationship with a physician or other professional. Please consult your
doctor for matters pertaining to your specific health and diet.

To contact the publisher, visit
www.createspace.com

To contact the author, visit
www.fabfertile.com

Printed in Canada

Cover photo credits: (top) Alena Ozerova/*Shutterstock.com*, (bottom
left) Yasonya/*Shutterstock.com*, (bottom middle) kohy/*Shutterstock.
com*, (bottom right) Yasonya/*Shutterstock.com*.

To Greg: I love you. You make the journey better every day.

CONTENTS

PART 1: FABULOUSLY FERTILE

PART 2: THE FABULOUSLY FERTILE

10-DAY CHALLENGE

ACKNOWLEDGEMENTS

To my graphic designer, Khamis Design Inc, Ali Khamis and Lynn Brenner for their amazing book cover and always delivering on a tight deadline.

Thanks to Mike Lalich for a great headshot and for making me feel so relaxed.

To Heather Andree for making my hair look great and to my makeup artist Kerry Schreman, thank you for making look like a better version of myself.

I would like to thank the ladies at the Burlington, BCBG, for the great wardrobe for my picture.

Thanks to all my manuscript readers Karen Spencer, Jo Davies, Karen Beattie, Carol Garrison, Margaret Leek, Alan Leek.

Thank you to Natalie Washington for your creativity and support with developing many of the recipes.

A special thank you to my editor Wendell Anderson.

I would also like to thank Dr. Shahnaz Chowdhury for supporting me and giving me the inspiration to write this book. This was my story all along, and not until I met you was I able to bring it to light.

Thank you to Lindsay Smith and Joshua Rosenthal for developing the Institute for Integrative Nutrition Launch a Book course. Your weekly encouragement and support made me dig deep and make the dream happen.

Thank you to my fellow coaches Dixie Lemke, Sherry Nash and Amanda Nahas Wilson. I believe we all need a coach to keep us on track. Thank you for your encouragement, words of wisdom and making sure I got out of my own way.

Thanks to my family. To Bruce Garrison for always being so positive and encouraging. To Carol Garrison for making me feel part of your family from day one and for always supporting me. To Dave Leek for always being there and for making me laugh with your twisted sense of humour. To Alan Leek for always believing in me and for giving me your entrepreneurial spirit. To Margaret Leek for inspiring me to be on this path and for pushing me to reach inside myself and bring out my voice. Your encouragement and unwavering support mean me so much to me.

To my extended family Dave, Reggie, Alison, David, McKenna, Dan, Molly, Isabel, Lisa, Jamie, Emma, Glenda, Paul, Matt, Ken, Nicole, Emily and Paige, thanks for your support. Jean and Jay Hooper, thanks for your encouragement and for showing my children such as good time at your horse farm.

To my ladies, what fun would it be without you? We've been friends for over 30 years. Debbie Van Grieken, Karen Beattie, Leza Kjarasgaard, Dawn Zontanos, Lea ann Donaldson and Rakiyah Mooynan. A special thank you to Karen Spencer for being my friend since I was 8 years old. I know I can always count on you.

To Ava, you inspire me every day with your beautiful spirit, go-getter attitude and warm generous heart. To Will, I love your natural self-confidence, your silly sense of humour and your kind, loving heart.

To my husband Greg, who listens to all my crazy schemes, keeps me laughing every day and supports me 100%. You make all this possible.

ABOUT THE AUTHOR

When Sarah Clark was 28 years old, she received a diagnosis of premature ovarian failure. She accepted the diagnosis and had both her children through in vitro fertilization. Years later she realized the root cause of her infertility was a food intolerance. As a graduate from McMaster University, a certified life coach with accreditation from the International Coaches Federation and a health coach with training from the Institute for Integrative Nutrition, she is deeply passionate about helping couples supercharge their fertility naturally. When she is not testing gluten-free and dairy-free recipes in her kitchen, she loves spending time with her husband and two children.

FOREWORD

A motivational guide that will empower and inspire all those couples who are struggling with infertility, to believe in their body's innate powers and rejoice hope.

Sarah was given the diagnosis of premature ovarian failure at the age of 28, and at that time her only option was IVF treatments. Today, even though IVF treatments continue to be the mainstream approach to attain pregnancy, couples are turning towards complimentary treatment options. Acupuncture, homeopathy, herbal medicine, nutraceuticals, Reiki, nutrition and lifestyle changes — just to name a few — are far more accessible and accepted today, and have shown to have immense benefits in conception.

In a society where diagnoses suppress hope, it was Sarah's quest and determination in finding the root cause of her infertility. In this journey, she was able to discover the power of food and significance of healthy lifestyle in nurturing one's soul, hence one's health. Unlike many fertility diet books that take a clinical approach, *Fabulously Fertile* inspires and enlightens people to take charge of their own health and well-being.

This book is very close to my heart, and I truly believe that it will nurture many lives and unfold them in positive ways.

Dr. Shahnaz Chowdhury, B.Sc., M.Sc., ND
Director of Halton Integrative Women's Health Centre
www.hiwhc.com

The Halton Integrative Women's Health Centre is Burlington, Ontario's, first multidisciplinary women's health centre. Our team specializes in a vast array of women's health concerns, with a special interest in fertility issues for both women and men.

MY STORY

In my early 20s, I always joked that I was having menopausal hot flashes. I would feel my whole body begin to flush, and the sweat would start dripping from my forehead. I thought I was prone to blushing. Little did I know that I was headed towards early menopause.

Slowly my periods began to disappear. At the time I really thought this was great, because I didn't need to deal with the monthly hassle. Then I began to experience other symptoms such as vaginal discharge, pimples on my previously flawless skin, dandruff and a small weird fungal rash on my chest. Yep, some pretty sexy stuff, but I didn't think it had anything to do with my fertility, so I didn't take the symptoms seriously.

Around the age of 27, many of my friends started having babies. I went to baby shower after baby shower and started to think that maybe it was time to start planning for a family. My life plan was always to get married at 25 (check, married my first love), have a baby at 28 and have a fabulous career too. Like many women, I wanted it all and didn't think anything would get in my way. We started trying right away, but nothing happened. I began to wonder why it was that I got my period only two or three times per year. Suddenly, my lack of periods became a major red flag. What was going on with my body? I didn't wait long until I consulted my family doctor and had my hormone levels tested. At the age of 28, I was diagnosed with premature ovarian failure. Premature ovarian failure is the loss of

function of the ovaries before age 40. I remember leaving my OB/
GYN's office with the in vitro fertilization brochure in my hand, in
shock, and not really sure what just happened.

After letting the news sink in and discussing the options with
my husband, I immediately went into action. Looking back, I didn't
take any time to grieve or really listen to what my body was trying to
tell me. The signals were right in front of me. The weird health complaints — such as vaginal discharge, adult acne and the chest rash —
but I was not yet able to connect the dots. We decided to pursue the
in vitro fertilization (IVF) route and opted to use a donor egg. I ap-
plied to a number of local fertility clinics and was placed on a list and
began the long wait for a match. Since patience is definitely not one
of my virtues, this was excruciatingly difficult. During this time, I
began to stalk the mail delivery person, because the donor's information would come to us in the mail. I began to look at every woman
around me and wonder why it was so easy for her to get pregnant and
not me. Why had my body failed me? Not one time after my diagnosis
of premature ovarian failure did I think to question the diagnosis and
seek alternative treatment. It was not even on my radar. The experts
and specialists had told me I would be unable to get pregnant with
my own eggs. I fully accepted the diagnosis.

Finally, the donor profile arrived in the mail, about one year after we signed up. My husband and I reviewed the information and
felt it was a good match. The eggs were taken from the anonymous
donor, and three live embryos were implanted in me. We had two
more embryos saved for another child. Luckily, at the age of 30, I
got pregnant with our daughter on our first try. I was one of the
fortunate ones, and didn't have to endure years of fertility treatments. About a year after my daughter was born, we tried again
with the frozen embryos. Unfortunately, these embryos didn't take,
and we were placed on the list again for another donor. My son was
born three years after my daughter with a live embryo. We were so
thankful and grateful that, finally, our family was complete.

Fast-forward many years to when I was 40 years old. I was in a stressful job, trying to juggle career and family and not feeling like I was in the best place creatively or spiritually. I was constantly stressed and had this niggling doubt in the back of my mind that I was not living up to my full potential. Turning 40 for me was the fork in the road. What was I going to do with my life? At the time I thought it was to continue to climb the corporate human resources ladder — until I found coaching. I enrolled in a coaching program to coach in the corporate area. Little did I know that this life-coaching course would change the course of *my* career. I left the course with a plan to start my own business in the health and wellness field. I then enrolled in the health-coach training program at the Institute for Integrative Nutrition to further deepen my knowledge. What I didn't realize at the time was that this course would change my life and my family's life forever and help me discover the root cause of my infertility.

During this time, my health was definitely suffering. Although I could still function, my immune system was so low that I began to experience many chronic health complaints. The vaginal discharge was still there, chronic bladder infections (I became allergic to many different types of antibiotics) and chronic sinus infections (every cold I got, and I had a lot of them, turned into a sinus infection). I had frequent headaches, moodiness, brain fog and extreme fatigue. I didn't want to cry in the corner; I wanted to kick the corner. Arrggh!

After learning in the health-coaching course how food can affect our health and discovering a little-known fungus called candida, I finally decided to consider some alternative treatments. After taking a food sensitivity test with my naturopath, I learned I had candidiasis. Candidiasis is a serious overgrowth of the yeast *Candida albicans*. It was recommended that I eliminate sugar, gluten, caffeine, dairy and alcohol from my diet. I knew I would need to do something, but had no idea it would be so radical.

I decided to take the recommendations seriously, and since I usually do everything full on, I immediately eliminated the recommended foods. The first three or four days were the worst. I had a major sweet tooth and was dreaming of sugar everywhere. I didn't know what to eat. I thought of food constantly. It was one of the hardest things I have ever done, but once I got through the middle of the first week, it started to get easier.

My headaches disappeared, and I didn't feel like I needed to go to the bathroom every minute. My sinuses started to clear. After about one month on the diet, when I rechallenged dairy and gluten, I found they both aggravated my system. I would get sinus congestion, and my bladder would act up. As I continued to keep dairy and gluten out of my system, my skin cleared up, the dandruff went away and the chronic vaginal discharge was finally minimized. The diet also improved my seasonal allergies; my allergies to cats lessened as well. Who knew that what we put on our fork every day could have such a huge impact on our health?

I wanted to write *Fabulously Fertile* to help couples with their fertility. I am passionate to get the word out that simple dietary and lifestyle changes can have a huge impact on your fertility. It took me over 12 years to figure out that the root cause of my infertility was due to a food intolerance that caused an overgrowth of candida in my system, which lead to many other health issues. I don't have many regrets in life, but I wish I had questioned my infertility diagnosis and had considered other treatment options.

Let this book be your guide to help you explore and consider other options on your path to conception. This book is for you if you are preparing for IVF or if you have any of the following:

- polycystic ovarian syndrome (PCOS)
- endometriosis
- unexplained infertility
- hormonal imbalance

- high or low follicle stimulating hormone (FSH)
- low sperm motility and count
- luteal phase defect
- hypothyroidism

Western medicine definitely is part of the solution, as well as nutrition, naturopathic, chiropractic, acupuncture, massage, yoga and meditation. Let me show you how to take charge of your health so you can learn how to supercharge your fertility naturally.

If you would like more information about my fertility coaching programs, contact me at *sarah.clark@sesacoaching.ca*. It would be my honour to be your guide.

I am eternally grateful that science helped me conceive my daughter Ava and my son Will. They both light up my life.

Part 1

FABULOUSLY FERTILE

One

WELCOME TO
FABULOUSLY FERTILE

Congratulations for taking control of your fertility! When you take an active role in your health, you become the conductor of your own healing. In the beginning you may have many questions and concerns, which can be overwhelming. That's where I come in. I'm here to support you and guide you to supercharge your fertility naturally. As you begin you will learn to tap into your intuition and listen to your own body. You know your body best. So let's get started.

The Fabulously Fertile book offers you a 10-day challenge. The 10-day challenge includes delicious and easy recipes, including a meal plan. You will eat plant-based foods during the 10 days. Then you may add some animal protein as tolerated afterwards. (Unless you have candida, then you may need to add some animal protein such as turkey or chicken during the 10-day challenge). The recipes rely on simple ingredients; offer a variety of tastes — such as Mexican, Italian, Indian and Moroccan — and are not filled with hard-to-find ingredients (you will get acquainted with your local health food store), although you may discover some new delicious fertility superfoods such as chia seeds, kale and quinoa, or some old standbys such as walnuts and bananas. You will start to rebalance your hormones and clear out the toxins.

These meals will have tips for your specific type of infertility. You can refer to the "Types of Infertility" section and recommendations if you are unsure of your fertility. You can complete the program, by yourself or with a buddy (your partner or spouse is best!). It takes 90 days for an egg to renew itself, and the life cycle of sperm is 70 to 80 days. It's best to clear out the toxins for at least three months before trying to conceive. The 10-day challenge is only the beginning. Once you begin to tune in to your body and feel how food directly impacts your health, there is no looking back. If you require further support, my coaching programs are designed to make permanent changes to your health and fertility. They are uniquely customized to your specific fertility needs. They include customized meal plans and individualized life-coaching support.

You may have experienced years of infertility or simply want to get your body ready to have a baby by clearing out the junk and toxins. You may have been on the birth control pill for years, and have come off the pill, but you have become out of touch with your body and its cycles. You may already have a child and are experiencing secondary infertility. This can be equally as devastating as primary infertility, or even more so. Many couples experiencing secondary infertility may receive well-meaning comments such as, "Well, at least you already have one child." This can be heartbreaking as the dream of completing your family is put on hold. I know this feeling first hand. After my daughter was born and the frozen embryos didn't work, we were placed on the donor-egg list again. Once again we had to wait and hope that science would help us to have another child. The hardest part was to realize I had no control over the situation. The yearning and panic feeling that I needed another child to complete my family was stronger than ever. I felt powerless. This book will show you how to take back your power. Many men also feel powerless and alone in the face of infertility.

Male factor infertility plays an important role in the desire to have a family. Many times the focus is on the woman, while 40% of infertility is due to the male. An infertility diagnosis for men can be isolating, embarrassing, a blow to the ego (am I not virile enough to father a child?) and can lead to depression. Men typically do not talk to their friends about infertility, join support groups or online chat rooms or ask for emotional support, like women. Support is essential when going through infertility, as it can be stressful and draining. This book will help you to discover that simple diet and lifestyle changes can impact male fertility. Also to know that support is here for you and that you are not alone. You will learn to listen to your body and supercharge your fertility naturally.

The 10-day challenge will help you to tune in to your body again. I'm here to tell you that you can begin to take back your power! Our body whispers to us, and we can either listen or wait until our body begins to start shouting, usually in the form of disease or illness.

Each section of this book will have "From Your Coach," (that's me! You'll never be alone!) to help guide you and bring awareness to your thoughts and actions. You will find out how to take yourself off automatic pilot. You will discover strategies to help you bust through old habits and instill healthy new fertility-boosting habits. You will learn techniques to reduce your stress and how to be kind to yourself. You will discover which foods to avoid and which foods you need to boost your fertility.

What we put in our mouth directly impacts our health. For years I was eating all the wrong foods, and it directly impacted my fertility.

> *When you know better, you do better.*
> —Maya Angelou

After the 10-day challenge, you will definitely know better.

What Is Next?
First, we will learn about the different types of infertility.

Two

TYPES OF
INFERTILITY

B elieve me, I know. You want to get going as soon as possible. You are running out of time. You are done putting the dreams of having a family on hold. Still, you are not sure where to start. I have got you covered. This chapter is for you. I know there is a lot of research and statistics, but don't skip it, because it will help you figure out the best place to begin and will serve as your roadmap.

It includes a summary of infertility types, together with diet and lifestyle recommendations. We will go into depth later in the book with regard to each dietary and lifestyle recommendation. Let this be your overview. Refer to this chapter often as you learn more about the tools needed to supercharge your fertility naturally.

Infertility can be a devastating diagnosis. There can be feelings of shame, guilt, worthlessness and social isolation, and difficulty concentrating or sleeping. And there can be anger and depression. It can put a major strain on a marriage as month after month the hope of completing your family is put on hold. Many couples struggle with infertility for years. This can lead to stress, which also greatly impacts fertility. Take a few moments to honour your journey. Honour where you have been and where you are going. It's time to begin to love yourself and practice self-compassion. Know that you are absolutely amazing. Take a slow, deep breath, and let that sink in. You are not alone, and support is all around you. Your infertility diagnosis does not have to define you; you can take back your power.

First, let's figure out how different types of fertility problems respond to natural treatment methods. In Canada one in six couples experience infertility. This number has doubled since the 1980s. Infertility is the inability to conceive after one year for women under 35, or six months for women over 35 years of age.[1]

According to Health Canada, the causes of infertility in women include:

- age (Fertility decreases after age 35.)
- problems producing eggs because of missed periods/menstrual cycle or no regular cycle
- having sexually transmitted infection such as chlamydia, which can cause blockages in the fallopian tubes
- problems in the uterus such as fibroids or polyps
- problems with the fallopian tubes such as missing tubes or blockages
- endometriosis (excess of tissue that gathers around the reproductive organs)
- hormonal imbalances
- early menopause (before age 40)

The causes of infertility in men include:

- poor sperm quality (their rate of movement and shape)
- low sperm count or lack of sperm
- a history of sexually transmitted infection such as chlamydia
- hormonal imbalances

Causes of infertility in both men and women include:

- past treatments for cancer (chemotherapy, radiation or surgery)
- some chronic illnesses such as diabetes, as well as their treatments
- tobacco and alcohol use
- being underweight or overweight

Female Infertility

For many women who experience problems with their period or hormonal imbalance, the general recommendation is to take the birth control pill to regulate their cycle. This will chemically regulate the system, but any underlying issues will always come back. When you are ready for conception, there is often a smaller window to balance the hormones to conceive. It's a better idea to balance the endocrine system now rather than covering it up with a daily pill.

Many women put their family on hold to pursue their careers. As a career woman, I get it. But often we start trying for a family and run up against an infertility diagnosis. This can be heartwrenching as the years start to tick by and we are unable to conceive. If you are in a time crunch and your fertility window is starting to close, these recommendations will get you started to supercharge your fertility naturally. You may have to slow down. (It's impossible to do it all and have it all — I know this first hand.) You will learn to practice some self-care and love. As you start to practice compassion towards yourself, you will begin to feel the stress and pressure slowly start to lift. You can take charge now; you no longer have to wait.

Also, you may be able to get pregnant, but are unable to carry the baby to term. Miscarriage is devastating and heartbreaking. You may experience a roller coaster of emotions and go through the stages of grief, starting with shock and denial, anger, guilt, depression and finally acceptance. Do not minimize these feelings, as they are complex and completely normal. It is important to enlist the support of your partner, friend, coach or therapist.

Here is a list of some of the more common female infertility types.

Polycystic Ovarian Syndrome

Polycystic ovarian syndrome (PCOS) affects 5% to 10% of women in childbearing age. There are a variety of symptoms, including absent or irregular menstruation, acne and excessive facial hair.

According to the PCOS Awareness Association, women with PCOS typically have high levels of androgens, missed or irregular periods and many small cysts in their ovaries. Women with PCOS are four times more likely to have a miscarriage due to the imbalance of insulin levels, as the embryo is unable to attach to the uterus.[3]. This is mainly due to obesity, which is commonly associated with PCOS.

PCOS is often precursor to type 2 diabetes and will benefit from changes to diet[4]. By reducing simple carbohydrates and sugar, insulin levels will decrease and the symptoms of PCOS will start to improve.

Foods to Avoid

- gluten (three months) white breads, cookies, pastries (simple carbohydrates that contain trans fat and chemicals)
- dairy (three months)
- soy
- fish containing high levels of mercury such as shark, swordfish, king mackerel and tilefish
- sugar, caffeine and alcohol
- starchy vegetables such as potatoes, corn and peas

Foods to Add

- whole grains such as gluten-free quinoa, brown rice and buckwheat
- low-glycemic-load fruits such as berries, apples and pears
- alternative sweetener such as stevia
- veggies such as kale, broccoli and asparagus
- legumes, nuts and seeds
- organic meats such as chicken and turkey
- fish such as salmon, trout, tuna and sardines

Additional Recommendations

- Try meditation or visualization.
- Throw out plastic.
- Aim for 30 minutes of nonvigorous exercise daily.
- Try acupuncture or massage.
- Take supplements: multivitamin, vitamin D.
- Take herbs and nutritional supplements: maca, vitex, tribulus terrestris, licorice root, natural progesterone cream, royal jelly, bee pollen, evening primrose oil.

Endometriosis

Endometriosis occurs when the tissue that lines the uterus (tissue called the endometrium) is found outside the uterus. This tissue can cover or grow into the ovaries or distort or block the fallopian tubes. This can lead to pain, irregular bleeding and problems getting pregnant. This causes fertility problems in about 30% to 40% of women.[5]

Symptoms include very painful cramps, heavy periods, chronic pelvic pain (which includes lower back and pelvic pain), intestinal pain, pain during or after sex, and infertility.[5]

Studies have shown that many women with endometriosis are intolerant to gluten.[6] It is best to avoid gluten and wheat for three months to determine if pain is reduced or eliminated. Many women with endometriosis are either intolerant to gluten or may have celiac disease.

Dairy consumption causes inflammation and congestion in the body, and dairy contains estrogen, which is inflammatory to the system. Many women with endometriosis notice improvement in their symptoms when they eliminate dairy. Eliminate dairy for three months, and determine if there is improvement with symptoms.

One study found that women drinking two or more cups of caffeine from coffee per day were found to be twice as likely to develop endometriosis than other women.[7]

Studies have found that red meat and ham consumption is associated with endometriosis risk. One study found that women eating red meat seven times a week or more were more likely to have endometriosis than women who ate red meat three times per week.[8]

Soy is not the wonder health food that we once thought. Most soy is genetically modified and not organic. Soy is mildly estrogenic and can increase estrogen in the body, which may contribute to pain associated with endometriosis. Eliminate soy, and determine if there is any improvement with symptoms.

Endometriosis may also be linked to candida.[15] Follow the candida protocol.

Foods to Avoid

- gluten (three months) (simple carbohydrates such as white bread, cakes, cookies)
- dairy (three months)

- red meat, pork
- soy
- fish containing high levels of mercury such as shark, swordfish, king mackerel and tilefish,
- sugar, caffeine, alcohol

Foods to Add

- whole grains such as gluten-free quinoa, brown rice and buckwheat
- dark green vegetables such as kale, mustard greens, broccoli, avocado
- low-glycemic-load fruits such as berries, apples and pears
- legumes, nuts and seeds such as flaxseeds, chia seeds
- organic meats such as chicken and turkey
- fish such as salmon, trout, tuna and sardines

Additional Recommendations

- Avoid plastics.
- Use organic personal care products.
- Eat organic.
- Try meditation or visualization.
- Aim for 30 minutes of nonvigorous exercise daily.
- Try acupuncture or massage.
- Take supplements: multivitamin, probiotic, vitamin C, zinc, omega-3s.
- Take herbs and nutritional supplement: progesterone cream, bee pollen, maca.

Uterine Fibroids

These are growths of smooth muscle and connective tissue that grow on the wall of the uterus. They affect more than 50% of women and are the most common reason for major surgery.[9] Fibroids are thought to be estrogen dependent. When levels are high from pregnancy or the birth control pill, fibroids can grow. Symptoms include heavy or prolonged periods, bleeding or unusual discharge between periods, pain and bleeding during intercourse, swelling or lower abdomen and infertility.[9]

Foods to Avoid

- gluten (three months)
- dairy (three months)
- soy
- red meat
- fish containing high levels of mercury such as shark, swordfish, king mackerel and tilefish
- sugar, caffeine, alcohol

Foods to Add

- whole grains such as gluten-free quinoa, brown rice and buckwheat
- organic fruits and vegetables (Pesticides have estrogenic affect on the body.)
- apples, cherries, broccoli, cauliflower, Brussels sprouts (They support liver detoxification of estrogen.)
- dandelion greens, beets, carrots, artichokes, onions and garlic (They stimulate liver detoxification.)
- legumes, nuts and seeds

- organic meats such as chicken and turkey
- fish such as salmon, trout, tuna and sardines

Additional Recommendations

- Avoid plastics.
- Use organic personal care products.
- Eat organic.
- Stress reduction is essential. Try meditation or visualization, focusing on decreasing the growth and size.
- Aim for 30 minutes of nonvigorous exercise daily.
- Try acupuncture or massage.
- Take supplements: multivitamin, vitamin E, vitamin D.
- Take herbs and nutritional supplements: evening primrose oil, vitex.

Luteal Phase Defect

This occurs when the ovaries are not producing enough progesterone in the second half of the menstrual cycle. This is the phase between ovulation and the woman's period. During this phase, the lining of the uterus normally becomes thicker to prepare for a possible pregnancy. If you have a luteal phase defect, the lining of your uterus does not grow properly each month. This can make it difficult to become or remain pregnant[16] This could be the cause of repeated miscarriages and a smaller percentage of women with unexplained infertility.[14]

Foods to Avoid

- gluten (three months)
- dairy (three months)
- red meat

- fish containing high levels of mercury such as shark, swordfish, king mackerel and tilefish
- sugar, caffeine, alcohol

Foods to Add

- whole grains such as gluten-free quinoa, brown rice and buckwheat
- fruits and vegetables, foods rich in vitamin C (bell peppers, broccoli, strawberry, blueberries, cranberries, raspberries, papaya, oranges)
- walnuts, flaxseeds, coconut oil
- legumes, nuts, seeds
- organic meats such as chicken and turkey
- fish such as salmon, trout, tuna and sardines

Additional Recommendations

- Stress reduction is essential. Try meditation or visualization
- Aim for 30 minutes of nonvigorous exercise daily.
- Try acupuncture or massage.
- supplements: multivitamin, vitamin C, omega-3s, coenzyme Q10
- herbs and nutritional supplements: vitex, natural progesterone cream

Male Infertility

For men a fertility diagnosis can be heartbreaking. Men may feel it is an insult to their masculinity if they are unable to get their partner pregnant. The dream of continuing a genetic line and fathering sons can be put in jeopardy. Men may also experience loss of desire or erectile dysfunction as their masculinity is compromised. This affects their relationship with their partner, as men may feel they have let her down by not being able to provide a child. It is important to seek the support from your partner, friend, coach or therapist. There are steps to take charge and supercharge your fertility naturally.

Sperm Problems
About 40% of infertility is related to male factor infertility. Low sperm count can be caused by:

- electromagnetic frequencies (EMF) (Keep you cell phone out of your pocket.)
- stress (Stress impacts hormonal imbalance.)
- pesticides and hormones in foods (Pesticides mimic estrogen.)
- alcohol
- plastics (When heated, they release xenohormones that mimic estrogen.)
- tight underwear (Testicles need to be kept at a healthy temperature.)
- hot tubs/bike riding (Difficult for testicles to regulate to a healthy temperature.)

Other factors include obesity, which is associated with decreased testosterone, decreased insulin and erectile dysfunction. Sperm defects such as abnormalities in shape of sperm or ability to swim can delay or prevent conception. Some men have antibodies against their own sperm.[11]

Foods to Avoid

- gluten (three months)
- dairy (three months)
- red meat
- fish containing high levels of mercury such as shark, swordfish, king mackerel and tilefish
- soy
- sugar, alcohol, caffeine

Foods to Add

- Whole grains such as gluten-free quinoa, brown rice and buckwheat
- fruits and vegetables, dark leafy green vegetables
- selenium (Brazil nuts, nutritional yeast, onions, garlic, leeks)
- zinc (Brazil nuts, cucumbers, peas, carrots, sesame seeds, pumpkin seeds)
- legumes, nuts, and seeds
- organic meats such as chicken and turkey
- fish such as salmon, trout, tuna and sardines

Additional Recommendations

- Avoid plastics.
- Use organic personal care products.
- Avoid EMF. Keep cell phone out of pocket, and do not put laptop on lap.

- Eat organic.
- Stress reduction is essential. Try meditation or visualization.
- Aim for 30 minutes of nonvigorous exercise daily.
- Try acupuncture or massage.
- Take supplements: multivitamin, zinc, vitamin C, folic acid, coenzyme Q10
- Take herbs and nutritional supplements: panax ginseng, maca, tribulus terrestris, ashwagandha.

Unexplained Infertility

About 20% to 25% of cases of infertility are unexplained infertility. This can be frustrating and confusing. Unexplained infertility can affect both men and women. The best place to start is with the diet.

Foods to Avoid

- gluten (three months)
- dairy (three months)
- soy (Eliminate for three months under the guidance of your healthcare practitioner if currently consuming two or three soy products per day. If not consuming soy, add for three months, but only after eliminating gluten for three months.)
- red meat
- fish containing high levels of mercury such as shark, swordfish, king mackerel and tilefish
- sugar, caffeine, alcohol

Foods to Add

- whole grains such as gluten-free quinoa, brown rice and buckwheat
- organic fruits and vegetables
- legumes nuts and seeds
- organic meats such as chicken and turkey
- fish such as salmon, trout, tuna and sardines

Additional Recommendations

- Avoid plastics.
- Use organic personal care products.
- Eat organic.
- Stress reduction is essential. Try meditation or visualization.
- Aim for 30 minutes of nonvigorous exercise daily.
- Try acupuncture or massage.
- Take supplements: multivitamin, omega-3s, coenzyme Q10
- Take herbs and nutritional supplements: panax ginseng (men), vitex, tribulus terrestris, maca

Hormonal Imbalance

Hormonal imbalance may be caused by a multitude of reasons, but the basic reason is an imbalance between progesterone and estrogen levels in the women's body. The pill and hormone replacement therapy (HRT) can cause hormone imbalance in the body. For men the hormonal imbalance may be an imbalance of testosterone, estrogen and progesterone. Both men and women are affected by cortisol, which is released upon stress.

Foods to Avoid

- gluten (three months)
- dairy (three months)
- red meat
- fish containing high levels of mercury such as shark, swordfish, king mackerel and tilefish
- sugar, caffeine, alcohol
- soy (Eliminate for three months under the guidance of your healthcare practitioner if currently consuming two or three soy products per day. If not consuming soy, add for three months, but only after eliminating gluten for three months.)

Foods to Add

- whole grains such as gluten-free quinoa, brown rice and buckwheat
- fruits and vegetables, especially dark leafy greens
- legumes, nuts and seeds
- organic meats such as chicken and turkey
- fish such as salmon, trout, tuna and sardines

Additional Recommendations

- Avoid plastics and other environmental toxins.
- Use organic personal care products.
- Eat organic.
- Stress reduction is essential. Try meditation and visualization.
- Aim for 30 minutes of nonvigorous exercise daily.

- Try acupuncture or massage.
- Take supplements: multivitamin, probiotic, omega-3s
- Take herbs and nutritional supplements: maca, evening primrose oil, royal jelly, bee pollen, ashwagandha, vitex, panax ginseng (men)

Follicle-Stimulating Hormone Levels

Follicle-stimulating hormone (FSH) is found in both men and women and is made by the pituitary gland. In women FSH is responsible for regulating the menstrual cycle and partially responsible for eggs in the ovaries. High levels indicate poor ovarian function, premature ovarian failure, polycystic ovarian syndrome or that menopause has begun. Low levels indicate eggs are not being produced and the pituitary gland may not be functioning properly. In men FSH controls sperm production. Too much estrogen or progesterone can cause FSH levels to be low. Ideal FSH level for pregnancy is under 10 IU/ml.[10]

Foods to Avoid

- gluten (three months)
- dairy (three months)
- red meat
- soy
- fish containing high levels of mercury such as shark, swordfish, king mackerel and tilefish
- sugar, caffeine, alcohol

Foods to Add

- whole grains such as gluten-free quinoa, brown rice

and buckwheat
- organic fruits and vegetables
- legumes, nuts and seeds, especially essential fatty acids (nuts and seeds)
- sea vegetables (wakame, kelp)
- organic meats such as chicken and turkey
- fish such as salmon, trout, tuna and sardines

Additional Recommendations

- Avoid plastics.
- Use organic personal care products.
- Eat organic.
- Stress reduction is essential. Try meditation or visualization.
- Aim for 30 minutes of nonvigorous exercise daily.
- Try acupuncture or massage.
- Take supplements: multivitamin, vitamin D, zinc.
- Take herbs and nutritional supplements: panax ginseng (men), vitex, maca.

Thyroid Problems

Hypothyroidism and hyperthyroidism can cause problems with fertility and miscarriage. Hyperthyroidism or hypothyroidism can cause male infertility, since sperm development requires normal thyroid levels.[12] Be sure to have your doctor check your thyroid. Some doctors may still flag your thyroid as normal when TSH levels are between 0.5 and 5.5 mIU/liter. Although recent data suggest that there could still be thyroid symptoms with TSH above 2.0 mIU/liter. One study found an increased risk of miscarriage if the TSH is above 2.5 mIU/liter in the first trimester[13]

Foods to Avoid

- gluten (three months)
- dairy (three months)
- soy
- fish containing high levels of mercury such as shark, swordfish, king mackerel and tilefish
- raw cruciferous vegetables (cabbage, cauliflower, spinach, Brussels sprouts, kale) (When eaten raw, they impede thyroid function. They can be eaten cooked.
- flaxseeds (may inhibit thyroid)
- sugar, caffeine, alcohol

Foods to Add

- whole grains such as gluten-free quinoa, brown rice and buckwheat
- organic fruits and vegetables
- foods with iodine (sea vegetables, strawberries, seafood)
- selenium (Brazil nuts, nutritional yeast, onions, garlic, leeks)
- zinc (Brazil nuts, cucumbers, peas, carrots, pumpkin seeds)
- legumes, nuts and seeds
- organic meats such as chicken and turkey
- fish such as salmon, trout, tuna and sardines

Additional Recommendations

- Avoid plastics.

- Use organic personal care products.
- Eat organic.
- Try meditation or visualization.
- Aim for 30 minutes of nonvigorous exercise daily.
- Try acupuncture (before and after treatments) or massage.
- Take supplements: multivitamin, zinc, omega-3s.
- Take herbs and nutritional supplements: panax ginseng, ashwagandha, licorice, maca, vitex.

If cleaning up your diet and adding the lifestyle recommendation does not work, you may still need to consider in vitro fertilization.

Preparing for in Vitro Fertilization
Prepare your body for IVF three months before your IVF treatment. Do not take any of the nutritional supplements or herbs once you begin treatment. Three months is suggested because the cycle of the egg is 90 days, and male sperm life cycle is 70 to 80 days.

Foods to Avoid

- gluten (three months)
- dairy (three months)
- red meat
- fish containing high levels of mercury such as shark, swordfish, king mackerel and tilefish
- sugar, alcohol, caffeine
- soy (Unless currently eating soy, then you may want to add it. Consult with your health practitioner.)

Foods to Add

- whole grains such as gluten-free quinoa, brown rice and buckwheat
- fruits and vegetables, dark leafy greens
- legumes, nuts and seeds
- organic meats such as chicken and turkey
- fish such as salmon, trout, tuna and sardines

Additional Recommendations

- Avoid plastics.
- Use organic personal care products.
- Eat organic.
- Stress reduction is essential. Try meditation or visualization.
- Aim for 30 minutes of nonvigorous exercise daily.
- Try acupuncture (before and after treatments) or massage.
- Try supplements: multivitamin, coenzyme Q10.
- Try herbs and nutritional supplements: maca, l-arginine, royal jelly, bee pollen.

What You Need To Know

- Gluten, dairy, sugar, caffeine and alcohol can be inflammatory to the body. Eliminate these to boost fertility.
- Do not consume red meat, as it decreases fertility in both men and women.
- Do not consume fish containing high levels of mercury such as shark, swordfish, king mackerel and tilefish.

- Gluten and dairy should be eliminated for three months to determine an intolerance and then rechallenged.
- A diet rich in whole foods, organic fruits and vegetables, free of environmental toxins such as plastics, is best for fertility.
- Stress-relief techniques are essential for fertility.
- Acupuncture is a good addition to your fertility-booting plan.
- Reach out for support from your partner, friend, coach or therapist.

From Your Coach
What thoughts come up when you think of preparing your body for fertility naturally? Skepticism. It's too hard to change your diet. Nothing has worked so far. Start to question those limiting beliefs. You may not have been successful so far, but the past is not a predictor of the future. Time to get curious about your thoughts without guilt or judgment. Write down your thoughts or share them with your partner, trusted friend or coach.

What may be holding you back?
Too busy? Fear or doubt? Not sure it will really work?

How have these thoughts served you in the past?
Remember, your thoughts and emotions are completely normal; it makes sense that you have fear, doubt and worry.

How can you turn these thoughts around and create a new more positive thought?
Try these thoughts: I am doing this program for me. I want to feel powerful and take a proactive role in my fertility.

Who will support you?
Partner, friend or coach.

Visualize your body being fueled with natural fertility boosting foods.
You feel clear of all toxins and junk. Your body is vibrant, healthy and strong. Set a clear intention for your journey. Commit to the program for three months.

What Is Next?
Time to commit and set your intention.

Handy Resources
Infertility Awareness Association of Canada
   http://www.iaac.ca/en/articles/blog
   The National Infertility Association, United States
   http://www.resolve.org/about/

References
1. *http://healthycanadians.gc.ca/health-sante/pregnancy-grossesse/fert-eng.php*
2. *http://www.womenshealth.gov/publications/our-publications/fact-sheet/polycystic-ovary-syndrome.html#b*
3. *http://link.springer.com/chapter/10.1007/978-1-4614-8394-6_15#page-1*
4. *http://www.sciencedirect.com/science/article/pii/S0026049514002108*
5. *http://www.sciencedirect.com/science/article/pii/S0026049514002108*
6. *http://europepmc.org/abstract/med/23334113*
7. Grodstein F, Goldman MB, Ryan L, Cramer DW. Relation of female infertility to consumption of caffeinated beverages. Am J Epidemiol. 1993;137:1353-1360.

8. Parazzini F, Chiaffarino F, Surace M, et al. Selected food intake and risk of endometriosis. *Hum Reprod.* 2004;19:1755-1759

9. *http://www.babycenter.ca/a7187/uterine-fibroids-what-you-need-to-know*

10. *http://www.advancedfertility.com/day3fsh.htm*

11. *http://umm.edu/health/medical/reports/articles/infertility-in-men*

12. *http://www.thyroid.ca/pregnancy_fertility.php*

13. *http://press.endocrine.org/doi/abs/10.1210/jc.2010-0340*

14. *uropepmc.org/abstract/MED/8005304*

15. *http://bodyecology.com/articles/find-out-what-this-widespread-reproductive-disorder-has-to-do-with-candida#.U-Y9NoBdWd5*

16. *http://www.webmd.com/infertility-and-reproduction/guide/luteal-phase-defect*

Three

SET YOUR INTENTION

We now know the diet and lifestyle recommendations for the different types of infertility. It is time to commit to fueling your body with optimal fertility-boosting foods. This can be scary as you say good-bye to some of your favourite foods, but you will begin to embrace delicious, energy-boosting, fertility-supercharging foods. This is where the rubber meets the road. It's time to go from talking the talk to walking the walk. Remember, you are not alone, and you are doing this for your future family.

Before we get started it's time to set your intention.

What is your dream for your body and your health?
Take a few minutes to visualize how your body will feel, how abundant and fertile you will become (if it helps, picture the fertility goddess). Visualize being full of vibrant healing energy.

How much effort are you willing to put in to get the result you are looking for? What can stop you or hold you back?
Sometimes we have limiting beliefs about a story we have made up in our head that we think is true. It's time to question those limiting beliefs and release the hold they have on you.

Some examples of limiting beliefs include:

- I have no willpower. (When you are committed, you will find a way.)

31

- Healthy foods don't taste good. (I'll show you that one isn't true.)
- I don't have the time to focus on my health. (If not now, then when?)
- The doctors told me it's not possible to conceive. (Time to add natural and alternative therapies to your toolkit.)

What has worked for you in the past and how can you leverage those strengths to propel you towards success?

Write your intention down in your food journal/diary. Refer to it daily. Writing it down helps to keep you accountable. This part is key.

There will be times when you may feel like you want to give up. Making changes to your diet and lifestyle is difficult. Remember, you will be excited in the beginning. During the second week, you may start to question your intention. This is completely normal. Make sure you have your support system in place before you begin.

When you make a commitment, it takes resolve and persistence. Refer to your intentions often to keep you on track. The more you bring awareness to your thoughts, the better able you are to deal with them.

Place your intention in a spot that you can see every day. Refer to it often throughout the day. This will keep you on track and strengthen your resolve.

What Is Next?

We live in a fast-paced world with many demands. How can stress impact our fertility?

Four

STRESS

Did you set your intention? If not, grab a piece of paper or your computer and write it out. Don't skip this step. OK, let's get started. What about stress? Many women don't give a second thought to getting pregnant. They are more worried about preventing pregnancy. This can be frustrating for couples struggling with infertility. The negative pregnancy test month after month can lead to feelings of failure and loss of control. When you are stressed, cortisol is released, which can impact ovulation. For men stress can affect the relationship with their partner, which lowers sex drive and desire for sex and can lead to erectile dysfunction. These feelings all contribute to high stress. Unfortunately, this becomes a vicious circle, because stress affects fertility.[1] This news may make you more stressed out and anxious. Take a deep breath, and slow down for a minute. You'll learn some coping strategies to reduce your stress. You can eat all the healthy food in the world, but if you are highly stressed, you may still be unable to conceive.

Research indicates that most cases of infertility can be attributed to a physiological cause in the man or woman. About one-third of the time, a physiological problem is identified in the woman, one-third of the time in the man, and about one-tenth of the time in both partners. In another 10% to 20% of cases (estimates vary), the basis of infertility cannot be determined.[2]

Another cause of stress is the decision to use IVF. You may be on edge and could be filled with worry about a positive outcome. I know these feeling firsthand. Although the clinic that I went to offered some counseling, it definitely was not enough to help me deal with the worry and stress associated with the procedure. I would have benefited from chiropractic care, acupuncture, yoga, meditation and having a coach to listen to me with a kind, empathetic ear. When you are going through IVF, there may be the added financial burden; the side effects of medication such as irritability, headaches or nausea; and the constant worry of a positive pregnancy result. These can be very stressful for couples and put a strain on a marriage. It is crucial to keep an open line of communication with your partner. Also realize that each partner may handle the stress of infertility differently and to respect and show compassion for each other's needs.

It is important to be kind to yourself and know that infertility can be heartbreaking, but that there still is hope. This is a time to learn to set boundaries and to make sure you have time for yourself. Figure out how many times during a day you are saying no versus saying yes. It's OK to say no to some things. It may be difficult to put your self first, but this is essential. Make sure that have you a support system in place. If you need support, ask your partner or a friend, or enlist the help of a coach or a therapist.

Learning to practice self-love and acceptance will help to reduce the feeling of stress and overwhelm. Begin by honouring the unique qualities in yourself and others. You may have lost touch with your intuition. Slowly start to trust yourself again and listen to your gut. Start to show compassion for yourself and others by caring for your body, mind and soul.

When you begin to love yourself and realize that putting yourself first is not selfish, but essential to your health and well-being, you can begin to make small steps every day to honour this commitment.

In times of stress, the best thing we can do for each other is to listen with our ears and our hearts and to be assured that our questions are just as important as our answers.

—Fred Rogers

Types of Stress Relief

There are many types of stress relief to consider. Find one that resonates with you.

Meditation is one of the simplest forms of stress relief and doesn't require much to get started. It is the concentrated focus upon a sound, object, visualization, the breath, movement or attention itself in order to increase awareness of the present moment. It helps to reduce stress, promote relaxation, and enhance personal and spiritual growth.[9]

Yoga is great stress-relieving tool and can boost fertility. Yoga can be helpful to reduce insulin resistance for women with PCOS. Yoga helps with the anxiety, and dealing with infertility can be very stressful. It is important to stay away from the more vigorous forms of yoga such as Ashtanga and power yoga.

Acupuncture is effective for stress management and to improve fertility. It has been around for more than 2,500 years. "Acupuncture is an ancient form of Chinese medicine involving the insertion of a solid filiform acupuncture needles into the skin at specific points on the body to achieve a therapeutic effect. Acupuncture is used to encourage natural healing, improve mood and energy, reduce or relieve pain and improve function of areas of the body".[8] Acupuncture has been shown to raise estradiol levels and help with menopausal symptoms such as hot flashes.[4] Acupuncture also helps women with PCOS to induce regular ovulation. It also helps to reduce the symptoms of PMS.[5] Receiving acupuncture on the day of embryo transfer significantly improves the reproductive outcome of IVF.

Chiropractic care is great for high stress. Chiropractors are nervous-system specialists. Reducing interference in the nervous system is their primary goal. They will help with fertility issues associated with improper nervous system function, poor nutrition, and poor lifestyle habits.[6]

Deep breathing: Try Dr. Andrew Weil's deep-breathing technique. This is a sure stress buster. Look to see how young children breathe — from their belly, not their chest. See Handy Resources at the end of this chapter for more details.

Progressive muscle relaxation helps to relax muscles by first tightening and then relaxing muscles throughout the body. Often we are unaware how tight our muscles are until we consciously relax them.

What You Need to Know

- Stress affects ovulation and lowers sex drive in men.
- Stress and the psychological impact affect fertility for both men and women.
- Learn to love yourself and be kind to yourself. Know that you don't have to do it all and that infertility can be extremely stressful and heartbreaking.

- Select a stress-relief technique that works for you. Meditation, guided visualization, chiropractic care, yoga and acupuncture are all good techniques.

From Your Coach
What comes up for you when you think of your stress levels?
You are so stressed, worried, anxious you don't know what to do, or you may feel numb and out of touch with your feelings. Maybe you are using a coping mechanism such as overeating, shopping or drinking to take your mind off your problems. Time to get real with yourself. Remember, no judgment; get curious with your thoughts. Grab a journal and start writing. Don't edit just let it flow.

What strengths have you used in the past to keep calm and feel relaxed?
Was it deep breathing, yoga or playing a favourite sport? Tap into your intuition. You know what works best for your body, mind and spirit.

How much time do you set aside each day to be quiet?
You are a human being, not a human doing. Time to get quiet.

What comes up for you when you think of meditation or visualization?
Sometimes people think they can't meditate because they can't sit still or their mind never stops. What if this one act gave you the peace of mind you need?

Who will support you?
Partner, friend or coach.

Visualize your favourite place in the world.
Maybe it's your cottage, a favourite vacation or walking in nature. Close your eyes, and let yourself feel completely secure, loved, calm and relaxed. Revisit these feelings when you want to feel at peace and calm.

What Is Next?
Could your daily personal care routine affect your fertility?

Handy Resources
Andrew Weil's breathing exercise
http://www.drweil.com/drw/u/ART00521/three-breathing-exercises.html
Information on progressive muscle relaxation
http://www.amsa.org/healingthehealer/musclerelaxation.cfm
Circle and Bloom: This site offers visualization and meditation programs specifically for fertility and pregnancy for both men and women. The programs include relaxation and guided visualization techniques to reduce the effects of stress and feel better about where you are on your family-building journey.
http://www.circlebloomcd.com/
Health Journey: Guided imagery for enhancing fertility. Includes calming and restorative affirmations and imagery to help with the ups and downs of fertility treatments and reclaiming one's life.
http://www.healthjourneys.com/Store/Products/Help-With-Fertility-Health-Journeys/89
Calm: Guided, timed meditation with calming music, babbling brooks and pictures of the sun setting. This can be accessed on your desktop. Available for free.
www.calm.com
Do Nothing for 2 minutes: Watch as the sun sets, and listen to waves crashing. If you touch your keyboard during the two minutes, a big "FAIL" comes up and the timer starts again.
http://www.donothingfor2minutes.com/

Buddhify: Packed full of guided meditation, this app has a timer to meditate without guidance. It also includes stats to see how you are doing. It helps you to grow your mindfulness.

www.buddhify.com

Oprah and Deepak Chopra Guided Meditation: Periodically they offer free 21-day guided meditation challenges. These meditations are then on sale after the free period is over. They have guided meditation on perfect health, desire and destiny, miraculous relationships and expanding your happiness.

https://chopracentermeditation.com/

Heartmath: Based on 23 years of research, Heartmath offers free programs for meditation, anxiety, stress, burnout and fatigue (just to name a few).

http://www.heartmath.org/free-services/solutions-for-stress/index-of-all-solutions.html?submenuheader=5

The Gifts of Imperfection: Let Go of Who You Think You Are Supposed to Be and Embrace Who You Are, a book by Brene Brown: This is one of my favourite authors. She has studied vulnerability, courage, worthiness and shame. Her no-nonsense approach is both highly relatable and laugh-out-loud funny.

http://www.amazon.com/Bren%C3%A9-Brown/e/B001JP45BA

References

1. *http://www.sciencedirect.com/science/article/pii/S1521693406001611*
2. *http://www.health.harvard.edu/newsletters/Harvard_Mental_Health_Letter/2009/May*
3. *http://informahealthcare.com/doi/abs/10.1080/1369713041000171 3814*
4. *http://informahealthcare.com/doi/abs/10.1080/j.1600-0412.2000.079003180.x*
5. *http://link.springer.com/article/10.1007/s00404-001-0270-7*

6. *http://americanpregnancy.org/infertility/infertilityandchiropractic.html*

7. *http://www.fertstert.org/article/S0015-0282(06)00212-3/abstract*

8. *http://www.afcinstitute.com/AboutAcupuncture/HowAcupunctureWorks/tabid/74/Default.aspx*

9. http://medical-dictionary.thefreedictionary.com/meditation

Five

ENVIRONMENTAL
TOXINS

Now that we are all Zen from our stress-busting meditation and visualization exercises, let's talk about those nasty environmental toxins. Time to throw out those plastic containers, rethink your personal care routine and start buying organic. These items are filled with environmental toxins that may be impeding your fertility. It could be the Bisphenol A (BPA) from your plastic bottle leaching xenoestrogens (chemical that mimics estrogen; *xeno* means "foreign") into your system. From the chemicals in your favourite skin care product to the lining of the cans that hold your food and many other kinds of plastic, xenoestrogens wreak havoc on women's hormonal system and men's sperm count.[1]

BPA has been shown to disrupt estrogen receptors.[2] Studies have shown that BPA prevents the embryo's ability to attach to the uterine lining and impedes the chances of successful IVF. [7] Plastics in baby bottles were outlawed only as recently as 2010 in Canada and 2012 in the United States. According to Environmental Defense, more than 150 peer-reviewed scientific studies have found BPA linked to potential health effects, including breast and prostate cancer, decline in testosterone, attention deficit hyperactivity disorder and a wide range of developmental problems.[3] BPA is found in the metal liners of food cans (look for BPA-free liners) and in plastic food and beverage containers. The BPA can leach out of the plastic, especially if the container is subjected to heat. It's best to use to stainless steel or glass containers. There is a high risk of BPA

41

exposure for fetuses, infants and children around puberty. "Young children are especially vulnerable because endocrine disruptors affect how their bodies grow and develop."[4]

Many of us are blissfully unaware of the chemicals in our daily personal care items. As Gill Deacon, the author of *There is Lead in Your Lipstick, Toxins in Everyday Body Care and How to Avoid Them,* shares that the average woman walks out the door in the morning and has been exposed to approximately 127 different chemicals. Our daily beauty routine is creating a toxic mess in our body. The David Suzuki Foundation shares that many companies refuse to disclose their ingredients because of proprietary rights. There are as many as 3,000 chemicals used in fragrance mixtures, including phthalates, some of which are suspected endocrine disruptors. A single product can include a mixture of dozens or even hundreds of fragrance chemicals. Many of these unlisted ingredients are irritants and can trigger allergies, migraines and asthma symptoms. Synthetic musks are of particular concern; Environment Canada categorizes some of them as toxic.

Parabens are the most common preservatives used in cosmetics and are often used as unlisted fragrance ingredients. They are absorbed through the skin and are endocrine disrupters and may interfere with male reproductive functions. They are often found in shampoo, diaper creams and other baby care products.[5]

Phthalates are manufactured chemicals used in plastics and as a preservatives for fragrance. They disrupt hormones and can cause birth defects of male reproductive organs. You'll find phthalates in scented baby products like shampoos, lotions and baby powder.[5] In one study exposure to phthalates was associated with reduced fertility when defined as a response to IVF treatment.[6]

Genetically Modified Organisms

It is best to purchase organic, if possible, to avoid genetically modified organisms (GMO) foods and pesticides. Study after study indicates GMO foods are endocrine disrupters for both male and female fertility. The high price of organic foods can be a deterrent to some, but the high cost of medical expenses and health problems far outweigh the risk. Opt for organic grass-fed, pesticide-free, free-range meats and produce. Fish that is wild-caught and sustainable is preferred. Watch out for the most prevalent GMO crops such as soybeans, corn and potatoes.

In the *Fabulously Fertile 10-Day Challenge,* we learn how to be a food detective. The best advice is not to eat anything from a box, but when that is not possible, check your labels. Get to know what is in your food. If you can't pronounce it, if it has more than five ingredients or if it doesn't rot, chances are you don't want to use it.[8] This is the same advice for personal care items. It may say "natural" or "organic," but what are the ingredients on the label? This is known as "greenwashing." Greenwashing is a marketing ploy that deceptively promotes a product as environmentally friendly. Some companies spend more money on advertising than implementing business practices that minimize environmental impact.

So how do you protect yourself and others from all these chemicals? Take action today.

Sign a petition to change current legislation.

Bottom line: Start reading products labels and be aware of what you are ingesting and putting on your skin. Ignorance is bliss but knowledge is power. This information is especially important if you have unexplained infertility or hormonal imbalance.

What You Need to Know

- Watch out for products that contain chemicals such as BPA, phthalates and parabens. They have chemicals that imitate estrogen and cause disorders in the reproductive system.

- Drink your water from a glass or stainless steel bottle; never drink from a plastic bottle.
- Don't reheat or store your food in plastic containers.
- Start reading your labels. If the food has more than five ingredients, doesn't rot or your can't pronounce the ingredients, don't eat it.
- Consider switching to organic fruits and vegetables, organic, free-range meats and wild-caught sustainable fish.

From Your Coach
What are your thoughts on environmental toxins?
Do you think organic is a hoax and way too expensive, or is the potential for reproductive disruption give you pause for thought? Time to get curious with your thoughts. Remember, no judgment; grab your journal and start to write.

What may be holding you back from eliminating the environmental toxins?
It's too time consuming. You don't have time to shop for all these different types of products. You like your current personal care routine. Your cupboards are filled with plastic containers. It's too expensive to replace everything. You may even feel overwhelmed by all the decisions that need to be made. Remember, these thoughts and emotions are completely normal.

How will you eliminate the toxins from your environment?
Take one action step today to minimize your risk of toxins. It could be buying a stainless steel or glass water bottle or trying a new organic soap or throwing out those plastics containers. Commit to one step today.

Who can support you?
Partner, friend or coach.

Visualize a clean, toxic-free environment for you and your baby.
Envision a clean, natural environment filled with organic healthy foods and safe, nontoxic products.

What Is Next?
We learn about a little-known fungus present in our bodies and its impact on fertility.

Handy Resources
The David Suzuki Foundation lists the dirty dozen to watch out for.
http://www.davidsuzuki.org/issues/downloads/Dirty-dozen-backgrounder.pdf
Check out this site to see if a product/service is using greenwashing.
http://www.greenwashingindex.com/
Competition Bureau: Contact if you see a business that is not being truthful about advertising its product or service.
http://www.competitionbureau.gc.ca/eic/site/cb-bc.nsf/frm-eng/GHÉT-7TDNA5
Environmental Defense (for Canadians): Sign a petition to change current legislation on harmful chemicals.
www.justbeautiful.ca
David Suzuki Foundation: Sign a petition to change current legislation on harmful chemicals.*http://action2.davidsuzuki.org/fragrance-petition*
Environmental Working Group (for Americans): Sign a petition to change current legislation on harmful chemicals.
http://action.ewg.org/p/dia/action3/common/public/?action_KEY=2044&tag=201309CorsmeticsCorpActionCenter

The Campaign for Safe Cosmetics *http://org2.salsalabs. com/o/5500/p/dia/action/public/?action_KEY=13369*

Natural Production Association: help in reading labels

http://www.npainfo.org/NPA/Consumers/NPA/For_Consumers. aspx?consumers=1

Cosmos: help in reading labels

http://www.cosmos-standard.org/

USDA Organic: help in reading labels

http://www.ams.usda.gov/AMSv1.0/getfile?dDocName=STELPR DC5068442

References

1. *http://www.sciencedirect.com/science/article/pii/ S0015028202043893*

2. *http://www.sciencedirect.com/science/article/pii/ S0303720706002292*

3. *http://environmentaldefence.ca/issues/banning-bisphenol-bpa*

4. *environmentaldefence.ca/reports/toxic-nation-guide-bisphenol*

5. *http://environmentaldefence.ca/issues/baby/toxic-chemicals*

6. *http://www.sciencedaily.com/releases/2013/07/130708103428.htm*

7. *http://www.washingtonpost.com/wp-dyn/content/arti- cle/2008/11/13/AR2008111303289.html*

8 *http://www.webmd.com/food-recipes/ news/20090323/7-rules-for-eating*

Six

CANDIDA

Now that we know how environmental toxins can impact fertility, it's time to turn our attention to candida. Many people that suffer from fertility problems have candida. *Candida albicans* is one of the many types of fungi that live in the intestinal tract. It shares the space in your bowel with a variety of other microorganisms, mostly friendly bacteria called "probiotics." Normally, candida causes no harm. However, antibiotics, high consumption of sugar and allergies can cause the friendly bacteria to die, leaving candida free to grow in parts or all through the body.[1]

My food intolerances to gluten and dairy led to the candida overgrowth in my system. I believe this was the root cause of my infertility. Looking back, if I had consulted an alternative health practitioner and changed my diet, I may have been able to become pregnant. This is something I will never know for sure. What I do know for sure is that diet and lifestyle changes have a direct impact on fertility. Depending on how long you have had candida, it may not be eradicated easily. It took me at least one year to get my body fully back on track; however, this varies for each person. Stress is a root cause of candida, so be sure to practice the stress-relief techniques. Be kind to yourself as you start to remove foods that may be contributing to the candida.

Although many conventional doctors do not recognize candida, it is linked to endometriosis, fibroids and ovarian cysts. It also may be linked to low sperm counts and motility issues with men. It can create a hormonal imbalance in your body. A candida waste product produces a false estrogen, and the body thinks it has produced adequate estrogen levels. This signals a reduction in its own estrogen. This can lead to infertility. Candida can also be transferred to your partner during sexual intercourse. For optimum health, each partner should follow the list of foods to add and avoid. *The Fabulously Fertile* 10-day challenge will get you started.

Take this quiz to determine if you may have candida.
http://bodyecology.com/quiz.php

If you think you may have candida, there are a number of tests that you can take. These tests can be helpful. Some people like to have a paper with a clear diagnosis. Often with candida the results can be inconclusive or the test may come back negative, even when you are exhibiting symptoms. Something to remember is that the gold standard to eradicate candida from your system is an elimination diet. Take out the foods that cause you inflammation in the body and then rechallenge the foods one by one. The 10-day challenge will eliminate the main foods that cause most people problems. Here are some tests to consider.

Testing Techniques
The following tests help to determine if candida is present in your system.

Saliva spit test: This can be done at home first thing in the morning. Spit into a glass of water. If the spit has projections moving downward in the water or becomes cloudy, this is a positive sign for candida. See Appendix A for more details.

Electrodermal screening: You can usually get this test through your naturopath who uses a noninvasive probe placed in your hands or feet.

These points correspond to acupuncture points. You receive a detailed report with tolerance levels for each food. See more in Appendix A.

Blood test: This test must be ordered through your physician. See Appendix A for more details.

Stool test: This test must be ordered through your physician. See Appendix A for more details.

Urine tartaric acid test: This test detects tartaric acid. The only source of tartaric acid is yeast. This test must be ordered through your physician.

Food Recommendations

- Eat more fresh vegetables, including low-glycemic fruits such as strawberries, blueberries, blackberries, raspberries, Granny Smith apples and pears.
- Eat whole grains (gluten-free).
- Avoid dairy, and instead drink nondairy milk such as coconut milk.
- Eat quality sources of lean protein such as beans and lentils (avoid for the first three to four weeks, and then reintroduce as tolerated), chicken, turkey and fish.
- Use stevia as a sweetener.
- Vegetable and green drinks will improve your resistance.
- Drink at least eight glasses of water daily to flush out the yeast toxin.
- Consume 1 to 2 tablespoons of ground flaxseeds daily. Flaxseeds have antifungal properties.

- Consume a daily probiotic and/or sauerkraut such as Bubbies.
- Take 1 tablespoon of unpasteurized apple cider vinegar mixed with a glass of water.

Foods to Avoid

- sugar and alcohol (The candida fungus feeds on sugar and yeast, so these must be avoided.)
- yeast in products such as bread, crackers and baked goods (You can request yeast-free breads at most gluten-free bakeries.)
- high carbohydrate foods: potatoes, corn, peas, squash, and sweet potatoes; and legumes such as chickpeas, black beans, azuki beans, lima beans, kidney beans, pinto beans and split peas (Avoid for the first three to four weeks, and then reintroduce as tolerated.)
- dairy
- foods with mold (nuts, nut butter) and mushrooms
- fruit juice, dried fruit and high-glycemic-load fruits such as tropical fruits, melons, oranges and grapes (It is especially important to avoid these foods between meals.)
- honey and maple syrup

Many people with candidiasis may also have food allergies. *The Fabulously Fertile 10-day Challenge* will help you to determine if you have an allergy. When you finish the 10-day challenge, you will need to introduce each food group back into you diet, or you can wait three months to reintroduce the foods. The choice is yours. When you rechallenge the food, wait three days before you introduce another food group back into your diet. For example, you could start with gluten and then try dairy. Journal how you feel, for example, indigestion, rashes, congestion, moods.

Watch out for die-off symptoms from the candida. Depending on the severity of your candida symptoms, you may want to consult your health practitioner to determine the best strategy to change your diet. Usually, the die-off symptoms last about one week and could include nausea, headache, chills, fever (just to name a few). Ensure you plan time for rest during this phase.

> *The definition of insanity is doing the same thing over and over again and expecting different results.*
> —Albert Einstein

Time to mix it up and start some new healthy habits.

What You Need to Know

- Candida may be the root cause of your fertility problems, and it may have caused a hormonal imbalance in your body.
- Take the quiz to determine if you have candida.
- Determine which test is the best fit for you to assess if you have candida overgrowth: saliva test, electrodermal screening, blood test, stool test or urine test.
- Review the list of food recommendations and the foods to avoid.

From Your Coach
What are your thoughts on candida?
It doesn't exist. I have never heard of it. Will healing my gut really help my fertility? Start to question those thoughts. Remember, no judgment; get curious with your thoughts. Grab a journal and start writing. Don't edit; just let it flow.

What are your thoughts on eliminating some of the top foods that aggravate candida?
It's too hard. I can't give up my sugar or sweet treat. What about the bread? My cravings are so strong, I'm always hungry. You may feel overwhelmed with all the changes you need to make. Remember, these thoughts and emotions are completely normal.

How will you eliminate the recommended foods and incorporate the new foods into your diet?
Take one small step today to eliminate one of the foods. Maybe you start with sugar, since sugar is fuel for candida. Remember you will experience withdrawal, so be kind to yourself and practice the stress-relieving techniques.

Who will support you?
Partner, friend or coach.

Visualize your body feeling strong, healthy and vibrant.
The candida has left your system, and your health and fertility are restored.

What Is Next?
How is your morning cup of Joe and daily pop habit contributing to your fertility problems? See how this daily habit could be affecting your fertility.

Handy Resources

The Body Ecology Diet: Recovering Your Health and Rebuilding Your Immunity by Donna Gates

Article on candida die-off

http://www.thecandidadiet.com/candida-die-off.htm

Article with good overview of candida

http://foodmatters.tv/articles-1/how-to-overcome-candida-naturally

References

1. *http://www.nationalcandidacenter.com/candida-what/*
2. *ww.webmd.com/skin-problems-and-treatments/guide/candidiasis-yeast-infection*
3. *http://www.wholeapproach.com/candida/symptoms.php*

CANDIDA: PROBLEMS, CAUSES, TESTS

Symptoms of Candida

Symptoms of Thrush[2]
Thrush is an infection of the mouth caused by the *Candida albicans* fungus.

- white patches on the inside of the mouth
- inflamed red patches on the skin
- bad breath
- heavily coated tongue
- dry mouth

Symptoms of Yeast Infection[2]
A vaginal yeast infection is an irritation of the vagina and the vulva. The yeast infection is caused by the Candida albicans fungus. In men the yeast infection can infect the penis, and usually affects men who are uncircumcised.

- vaginal itching, pain and burning
- thick yellow discharge
- red rash on penis
- itching or burning on the tip of penis
- burning during urination

Symptoms of Systemic Candidiasis[3]

- constipation
- persistent fatigue
- rectal itching
- kidney and bladder infections
- diarrhea
- muscle pain
- colitis
- arthritis
- abdominal pain
- canker sores
- congestion
- cough
- headaches
- mood problems (depression, anxiety)
- numbness or tingling in limbs
- chronic skin rashes
- poor memory and concentration
- allergies
- genital and toenail fungus

Root Causes of Candida

- prolonged or frequent use of antibiotics or corticosteroids, leading to depletion of good bacteria
- allergies
- stress
- hormonal changes and birth control pills
- poor digestion and elimination
- a depressed immune system

- a high sugar diet
- aging

Testing Methods

Spit Test
The best time to do this test is the first thing in the morning as soon as you wake up. Before you rinse, spit or put anything in your mouth, get a glass of water (in a clear glass). Now build up a bunch of saliva (just mouth saliva; do not cough up anything), and spit it into the glass of water. Observe what happens.

The saliva will float. That is OK and normal. If within 15 minutes you see thin projections extending downward into the water, it is a positive sign for candida. The projections may look like hair or small strings, like a jelly fish or spider legs, moving down into the water from the saliva floating on the top. Other positive indications might be very cloudy saliva that will sink to the bottom of the glass within a few minutes or particles that slowly sink or suspend below the saliva glob. What you are seeing are colonies of yeast which band together to form the strings.[1]

Blood Test Genova Diagnostics and Great Plains Laboratory specialize in functional laboratory testing and offers an Anti-Candida Antibody test, an immunological test which evaluates blood for the immune response to *Candida albicans*. The blood test is the most reliable test to determine if you have candida. It may be taken in conjunction with the stool test for further reliability. Genova diagnostics has the Candida Intensive Culture that will test both stool and blood.

http://www.gdx.net/product/anti-candida-antibody-immunological-test-blood

http://www.greatplainslaboratory.com/home/eng/food_allergy_igg.asp

Electrodermal Screening

During EDS, a blunt, noninvasive electric probe is placed on the patient's hands or feet at specific points. These points correspond to acupuncture points, which are the beginning or end of energy meridians. Energy transfers its signal through an acupuncture meridian to the nervous system. Minute electrical discharges from the acupuncture points are measured and indicate the condition of the body's organs and systems. There is some controversy as to whether this testing works, but it is good for someone that needs to see the foods they must avoid. The test will also determine if there is candida.

Stool Test

Genova Diagnostics and Great Plains Laboratory offers a comprehensive stool analysis. The test will provide a comprehensive look at the overall health of the gastrointestinal tract and for levels of yeast and pathogenic bacteria. This test may not be as reliable as a blood test. Often candida does not show up on this test.

http://www.gdx.net/product/comprehensive-digestive-stool-analysis-cdsa

http://www.greatplainslaboratory.com/home/eng/stool.asp

Seven

CAFFEINE

You now know how candida can affect your fertility. Next, let's learn how caffeine is affecting your fertility. Caffeine wakes us up in the morning and keeps us going when we hit the 3 p.m. slump. Many of us are addicted and can't get through the day without our daily dose.

Did you know that your chances of getting pregnant decrease when you drink caffeine? One study found that women who consumed more than the equivalent of one cup of coffee per day were half as likely to become pregnant, per cycle, as women who drank less.[3] Another study found that high doses of caffeine intake during pregnancy increased the risk of miscarriage.[1] As well, caffeine delays the transit of the fertilized egg from the tube to the uterus.[7] Fibrocystic breast disease, PMS, osteoporosis, infertility problems, miscarriage, low birth weight and menopausal problems such as hot flashes are all exacerbated by caffeine consumption.

Caffeine is in more than just coffee. It is in energy drinks and colas. Noncola drinks such as root beer and orange soda have caffeine too. Sunkist orange soda has 41 milligrams of caffeine; that's more than Coke's 35 milligrams. Thought you were getting your healthy vitamin C? Think again.

The Nurses' Health Study (Harvard University conducted an eight-year study of more than 18,000 female nurses) found that caffeinated soft drinks were associated with a higher risk of ovulatory infertility among women consuming at least two or more caffeinated soft drinks per day. Women consuming two or more caffeinated soft drinks per day had a 47% greater risk of ovulatory infertility than women who consumed less than one caffeinated soft drink per week.[9] To be clear, the sugar may be to blame for the infertility rather than the caffeine, as the high sugar content in soft drinks spikes insulin levels and can lead to weight gain. The key is to be aware of how much caffeine you are consuming on a daily basis. Sometimes it's more than we think and in the form of chocolate.

Do you crave a little bit of chocolate? Go ahead and make the switch to dark chocolate, but be aware there is still caffeine present. A 1.5-ounce serving of 80% cacao dark chocolate can contain more than 40 milligrams of caffeine, with some more expensive brands having up to 75 milligrams.[4]

Don't get me wrong. There are some health benefits to caffeine consumption such as increased alertness, improved mood, more energy, better concentration and preventing disease such as Parkinson's disease and Alzheimer's.[8] However, to boost your fertility and get your body ready to conceive, it's time to select another drink of choice.

The key is not to quit cold turkey. This is not recommended! Go slowly. Caffeine withdrawal causes headaches, body aches, stomach problems, irritability, depression and fatigue. Here is your plan to quit coffee, colas and chocolate. You can wean yourself off caffeine gradually before you start *the Fabulously Fertile 10-day Challenge*, or you can reduce your intake during the 10-day challenge. The choice is up to you.

Your Plan to Quit Coffee

Days 1–4

- Drink 50% decaf with 50% regular coffee.
- Before your coffee, consume one glass of water with lemon.
- Drink one glass of water before every coffee that you drink.

Days 5–9

- Drink 75% decaf and 25% regular coffee.
- Continue to drink one glass of water with lemon before every coffee you drink.

Day 10

- Drink 100% decaf, or you may switch to caffeine-free herbal tea or water.

Your Plan to Quit Tea

- Follow similar protocol to coffee.
- Drink 50% decaf tea with 50% regular and so on.
- Reduce the time you steep your tea.
- Green tea still has caffeine, but it will help as you transition to caffeine-free herbal tea.
- Before every cup of tea, drink a glass of water with lemon.

Your Plan to Quit Pop And Energy Drinks

- Don't quit cold turkey.
- Drink 25% less the first week, 50% for the next week and so on.
- Make sure you drink one glass of water with lemon before each pop or energy drink.
- Make sure you drink enough liquid. If you were previously drinking five colas per day, make sure you

have at least five glasses of water per day, or you may find it hard to stop.

- Find an alternative to pop such as sparkling water or water with lemon or stevia.

Your Plan to Quit Chocolate

- Similar to coffee, tea, pop and energy drinks — don't go cold turkey.
- Switch to high-quality dark chocolate with at least 70% cocoa.
- Reduce to every other day on week two and two or three times per week on week three.[10]
- Try raw cocoa nibs. They can be quite bitter, but they have the magnesium and the chocolate high without the sugar and the fat of chocolate.

Motivation is what gets you started.
Habit is what keeps you going.
— Jim Ryun

It's time to start a new healthy habit around your caffeine addiction. Refer back to the intention you set at the beginning of the book. It will keep you going when the going gets tough. Practice self-compassion, and if you get too frazzled, you can always start again the next day.

Removing caffeine takes time for your system to adjust. If you do slip up and have some chocolate or coffee, don't feel guilty. Stop, pause and savour what you are eating. Take the time to eat and drink very slowly while savoring every bite or sip. Once you remove the guilt and shame around eating, you start to bring awareness to your thoughts, and you are able to change old patterns.

What You Need to Know

- Caffeine reduces the chances of becoming pregnant. Women who consumed one cup of coffee per day were half as likely to become pregnant.
- Fibrocystic breast disease, PMS, osteoporosis, infertility problems, miscarriage, low birth weight and menopausal problems such as hot flashes are all exacerbated by caffeine consumption.
- Do not quit caffeine cold turkey.
- Follow the steps to quitting caffeine gradually.

From Your Coach
What time of the day do you crave caffeine?
Morning? Afternoon? Night? Do you have it in a social setting, or do you use it as a reward? First bring awareness to your habits around caffeine. Once you bring awareness to your actions, you are no longer on automatic pilot. Habits don't dissolve over night. Remember to be kind to yourself. Time to get curious, no judgment. Grab your journal and start to write.

How do you feel just before you have the caffeine?
Tired? Wired? Jittery? Time to tune in to your body. If you are feeling tired, try going to bed and waking up at the same time every day. If you are feeling bored, stressed or lonely, try calling a friend or going for a walk instead of having the caffeine. Remember, these thoughts and emotions are completely normal.

What is one step you can take today to reduce your caffeine consumption?
You can start by having a glass of water before you have your coffee or cola. If you decide to have some caffeine, instead of gulping it down, take a few minutes with no interruptions and really savour the caffeine. How does it make your body feel?

Who will support you?
Partner, friend or coach.

Visualize how your body will feel when it is free of caffeine.
Envision feelings of being grounded, calm, alert, rested and peaceful.

What Is Next?
Could your daily serving of meat be affecting your fertility?

Handy Resources
Naked Chocolate: The Astonishing Truth About the World's Greatest Food by David Wolfe and Shazzie
   http://www.amazon.ca/Naked-Chocolate-Astonishing-Worlds-Greatest/dp/1556437315

References
1. *http://www.ajog.org/article/S0002-9378(0702025-X/abstract?cc=y=?cc=y=*
2. *http://www.sciencedirect.com/science/article/pii/S001502829800257X*
3. *http://www.sciencedirect.com/science/article/pii/S0140673688909336*
4. *http://www.livestrong.com/article/288379-does-dark-chocolate-contain-caffeine/*
5. 12 "Caffeine & Women's Health." Food Insight. N.p., 15 Oct 2009. Web. 22 Dec 2011.

6. *http://www.sciencedirect.com/science/article/pii/ S0002937801110276*

7. *http://onlinelibrary.wiley.com/ doi/10.1111/j.1476-5381.2011.01266.x/full*

8. The Highs and Lows of Caffeine Consumption, Institute for Integrative Nutrition

9. *http://www.ncbi.nlm.nih.gov/pmc/articles/PMC3071680/*

10. How to Stop eating Chocolate all the time - *http://www.wikihow.com/Stop-Eating-Chocolate-All-of-the-Time*

Eight

PROTEIN

Now you know the impact caffeine has on your fertility, and you think to yourself, "There is no way I'm giving up my steak too." For some of my clients, the biggest hurdle of the 10-day challenge is eliminating animal protein. It has been so ingrained into our culture that the only way to get protein is from animal products.

I grew up mostly vegetarian. My friends always made fun of my weird food. This was back in the early eighties when I took sardine, alpha sprouts and pita bread sandwiches to school for lunch. Although at the time I yearned to have my friend's lunch of Chef Boyardee and honey sandwiches, I now thank my mother for showing me how real food tastes. Over 20 years ago my parents made the transition to a vegan diet. This was when everyone was asking, "What's a vegan? What do they eat?" And the question that still gets asked today, "Where do you get your protein?" As my mom likes to explain it means, "I eat nothing with a face."

When I left home, I assumed the standard Western diet, and my health and fertility began to deteriorate.

According to the Harvard Nurses' Health Study, when you get more of your protein from plants and less from animals, you improve your chances of getting pregnant[1] In the study, women with the highest consumption of animal protein had 41% greater risk of ovulatory infertility than women who consumed more plant protein[2] The study found that adding one serving a day of red meat and chicken increased risk of ovulatory infertility.[2] One serving of eggs and fish did not influence ovulatory infertility.[2]

The Fabulously Fertile 10-Day Challenge focuses on a plant-based approach to fertility. The focus is vegetables, fruits, whole grains, legumes, nuts and seeds. (Unless you have candida, then you may need to add some animal protein such as turkey or chicken during the 10-day challenge). If you suffer from irritable bowel syndrome, colitis or Crohn's disease, or general digestive upset, exercise caution when introducing a mostly plant-based plan into your diet. Consult with your healthcare practitioner, as you may want to slowly introduce legumes into your diet to prevent further aggravation to your system. When you have finished the 10-day challenge, depending on your fertility requirements, you may add organic meat and fish as tolerated. As the research tells us, when you reduce your animal protein, you increase your fertility.

Many people become accidental vegetarians or vegans because they like how their body feels when they reduce or eliminate animal protein. The meals in the 10-day challenge are easy and delicious. Your cravings will disappear; you will have more energy; and the brain fog will lift.

Little did I know that this one change in my diet would be so impactful for my health. I definitely had no intention of eating more plants. I made fun of my mom for years for eating vegan and being all "health conscious." I thought she was denying herself all of life's pleasures. Little did I know that after reducing animal protein, my health would improve. I ate minimal red meat, but I consumed more animal protein than I actually realized. When I minimized my animal protein consumption, I began to have more energy and noticed that my digestion was running smoothly.

A common symptom of eating meat is constipation. The normal transit time for all foods in your system is 40 hours. For women it is 47 hours and for men it is 33 hours.[3] Foods sitting in you digestive system for a long period creates a breeding ground for viruses, bacteria and tumours. Diseases such as cancer, heart disease, diverticulitis, irritable bowel syndrome, obesity and arthritis have some link to constipation.

When you start introducing more plant-based foods into your diet, go slowly, as your digestion can be adversely impacted. To reduce gas and bloating, try Beano.

> *Most people are more comfortable with old problems than with new solutions.*
> —Author Unknown

We know that we need to reduce red meat, but switching to a mostly plant-based diet can be scary. What if this were the new solution that would have the greatest impact your fertility?

What You Need to Know

- Animal protein consumption increases the risk of ovulatory infertility by 41%.
- One serving of red meat and chicken per day increases risk of ovulatory infertility.
- Aim for at least half your protein from plants.
- Animal protein contributes to constipation, which is linked to many diseases, including cancer, obesity and heart disease.

From Your Coach
What are your thoughts on eating a plant-based diet?
Do you worry you will be hungry or not be satisfied? It is true that some people may feel better eating slightly more animal protein such as people with blood type O. However, the research is clear; reduced animal protein directly impacts fertility. Time to get curious with your thoughts. Remember, no judgment; grab your journal and start to write

What may be holding your back from reducing your animal protein consumption?
You don't how to get your protein. (I'll show you how with our delicious recipes.) You've tried beans and they are horrible. (I'll show you they can be delicious.) You can't imagine your meal without the meat. You may even feel overwhelmed by all the decisions that need to be made. Remember, these thoughts and emotions are completely normal.

What is one step you can take today to add more vegetables, whole grains and fruits to your diet?
When you add food to your diet rather than take food away, you can feel more satisfied than deprived. Eat one meal each day that is plant based. Start with a smoothie for breakfast or a salad with beans for lunch. Commit to one step today.

Who will support you?
Partner, friend or coach.

Visualize how your body will feel when you eat a mostly plant-based diet.
Envision your digestion running smoothly, your skin feeling supple and looking flawless, your body feeling lighter and with more energy.

What Is Next?
Discover how you favourite sweet treat may be impeding your fertility.

Handy Resources
The China Study by T. Colin Campbell: This book details the connection between nutrition and heart disease, diabetes and cancer. This is the book I turn to when someone questions the validity of eating a plant-based diet.

Forks Over Knives: A film Based on the findings of the *China Study*. Chronic and degenerative disease like heart disease, diabetes and cancer can be prevented and most of them reversed with food.

List of protein amounts in plants
http://foodmatters.tv/articles-1/top-6-plant-based-proteins
Eat Right for Your Blood Type by Peter D'Adamo
http://www.amazon.com/Eat-Right-Your-Type-Individualized/dp/039914255X/ref=sr_1_1?s=books&ie=UTF8&qid=1407681188&sr=1-1

References
1. *http://www.sciencedirect.com/science/article/pii/S0002937807008332*
2. *http://www.ncbi.nlm.nih.gov/pmc/articles/PMC3066040/*
3. *http://www.mayoclinic.org/digestive-system/expert-answers/faq-20058340*

Nine

SUGAR

You learned how animal protein could impact your fertility. Could your daily trip to the vending machine for a chocolate bar or your nightly cookie habit impact your fertility too?

You might not have heard this before, but sugar is toxic. It is highly addictive and causes us to gain weight, not fat. Studies have shown that sugar is eight times more addictive than cocaine.[3] We know sugar is in baked goods, ice cream and candy, but sugar is hiding in many of your favourite foods. Watch out for sugar in low-fat yogurt, Chinese takeout, ketchup, peanut butter, pasta sauce, just to name a few. Also watch out for juice. An 8-ounce glass of orange juice has 8 teaspoons of sugar, and an apple juice has 10 teaspoons of sugar. A coke has 12 teaspoons of sugar. Not the healthy morning drink that you thought. A good rule of thumb to figure out how much sugar in your food is 4 grams of sugar = 1 teaspoon of sugar.

The American Heart Association recommends that women consume no more than 100 calories per day from sugar and men take in no more than 150 calories per day. That is about 6 teaspoons per day for women and 9 teaspoons per day for men.[5] Did you know there are 19 grams, or 5 teaspoons, of sugar in a 4-ounce container of yogurt? That's almost your daily limit, and that doesn't include the sugar in your coffee, your daily chocolate fix or that late night run for ice cream.

Today, the average Canadian consumes 26 teaspoons of sugar per day. That's 40 kilos, or 88 pounds, a year, or the equivalent of 20 bags.[6]

We use sugar to get us going in the morning, in coffee to pick us up again during the midmorning break with a muffin or donut. Quitting sugar can be difficult, but the rewards are so great. The first two or three days you may experience headaches, cramps, dizziness, irritability and nausea. Eliminating sugar gradually will lessen the withdrawal symptoms. Without the sugar you may notice that moods begin to even out. Many of my clients tell me they didn't know how bad they were feeling until they changed their diet and began to feel amazing.

Problems with Sugar

Sugar increases our energy, but then our blood sugar drops and we are hungry again. Nearly everyone craves sugar. It is the body asking for energy. However, chronic consumption of sugar dulls the brains mechanism to tell us to stop eating.

Sugar creates a hormonal imbalance in the body. All the sweet treats we consume raise our insulin levels. This spike in blood sugar gives us that temporary high, but then watch out as our blood sugar plummets. This causes continued stimulation of the adrenal glands. The adrenal glands release cortisol and adrenalin in an attempt to raise sugar levels. When this happens repeatedly, the adrenals become weakened, and this may lead to hormonal imbalance. This creates a roller coaster ride in the body with blood sugar erratically rising and falling. The adrenals are responsible for maintaining a proper balance between DHEA, estrogen, testosterone and progesterone. This affects hormone levels for both men and women.

What about insulin resistance? The pancreas secretes insulin to control blood sugar levels. Excessive sugar consumption can lead to insulin resistance. Insulin resistance disrupts normal ovulation by preventing the body from ovulating. Insulin resistance can be blamed for problems with ovulation and higher risk of miscarriage.[1] Many women with PCOS have insulin resistance. Some 50% of women with PCOS will have diabetes or prediabetes before the age of 40.[4]

Sugar also causes inflammation in our body. Inflammation is the body's healthy response to injury and infection. However, chronic inflammation can lead to heart disease, cancer, arthritis and Alzheimer's. Sugar also unbalances our immune system. For women with endometriosis, removing sugar, refined foods, white breads and pastas helps with the pain of endometriosis. Sugar also is fuel for candida. The more sugar we eat, the more we fuel candida, and candida creates major cravings for sugar. It's a vicious cycle. If you have candida, you must eliminate all sugar including most fruit. (Follow the candida recommendations in chapter 6.)

How to Cut Down on Sugar

Since we are surrounded by sugar everywhere, what are we to do? First step is crowd out sugar with the good stuff. Load up on veggies, healthy whole grains, legumes, nuts and seeds. When you are stuffed with delicious salads, healthy baked goods and yummy snacks, it's hard to keep eating your usual sugar-laden treats. Eat small balanced meals every four to five hours.

Try some processed, sugar-free alternatives such as maple syrup, honey or stevia. If you have insulin resistance, diabetes or PCOS, stick with stevia, as maple syrup and honey are still high on the glycemic index, but still lower than sugar. The glycemic index measures how quickly a certain food raises blood sugar levels. Foods with a glycemic index of 55 or below are considered to be low-glycemic foods. Pure maple syrup has a glycemic index of 54, and sugar has a glycemic index of 65.

Here are some of my favourite sugar substitutes.[10]

Brown rice syrup: This product consists of brown rice that has been ground and cooked, converting the starches to maltose. Brown rice syrup tastes like moderately sweet butterscotch and is quite delicious. In recipes replace each cup of white sugar with ¼ cup brown rice syrup, and reduce the amount of other liquids.[7]

Honey: One of the oldest natural sweeteners, honey is sweeter than sugar. Depending on the plant source, honey can have a range of flavours, from dark and strongly flavoured to light and mildly flavoured. Raw honey contains small amounts of enzymes, minerals and vitamins. It's also said that consuming local honey can help build up your immunity to common allergens in your area by introducing your body to the bee pollen.[11]

Maple syrup: Maple syrup is made from boiled-down maple tree sap and is a great source of manganese and zinc.[8] Approximately 40 gallons of sap are needed to make 1 gallon of maple syrup. It adds a pleasant flavour to foods and is great for baking. Be sure to buy 100% pure maple syrup and not maple-flavoured corn syrup. Grade B is stronger in flavour and said to have more minerals than Grade A.

Stevia: This leafy herb — also known as honey leaf — has been used for centuries by native South Americans. The extract from stevia is approximately 100 to 300 times sweeter than white sugar. It can be used in cooking, in baking and as a sugar substitute in most beverages. Stevia has been shown to have a positive effect on blood sugar levels by increasing insulin production and decreasing insulin resistance.[9] Stevia is available in a powder or liquid form, but be sure to get the green or brown liquids or powders, as the white and clear versions are highly refined.

Like a good girl or boy scout it is important to be prepared. When you have healthy food options available, you are less likely to grab something sweet. This takes time in the beginning. Be kind to yourself. But once you start the new habit of making healthy snacks available, watch as your health starts to soar.

Here are few snacks to keep on hand when a craving hits.[12]

Trail mix: A custom blend of nuts (walnuts, cashews, macadamia), seeds (sunflower, pumpkin), dried fruit (dates, prunes, raisins), which offers a great protein boost. Do not eat nuts or dried fruit if you have candida.

Carrot sticks/crackers with hummus: A perfect blend of crunchiness and smoothness. Make your own hummus or find spiced varieties made without preservatives at your health food store.

Fruit: Apples, pears, strawberries, raspberries, blueberries, blackberries, pineapple. Slice apple/pear and dip with maple syrup, brown rice syrup, honey or nut butters (almond butter, cashew butter).

Corn chips with salsa: Organic corn chips with organic salsa make a quick snack.

Rice cake with nut butter: Spread nut butter (cashew, tahini) on these light crispy cakes.

Smoothie: Almond milk or nondairy milk (1-1/2 cup), blueberries (½ cup) hemp hearts (1 or 2 tablespoons), 1 tablespoon almond butter. Combine ingredients in blender.

Green juice: Romaine lettuce (whole head), celery (2 or 3 stalks), cucumber ½,
Granny Smith apple (quartered). Juice ingredients in a juicer.

Many times when you crave sugar, you are actually dehydrated. Try having a glass of water before you go for a snack, and see if your cravings disappear. Better yet, add some berries or lemon and limes to your water for a spa-like treat.

Removing sugar from your diet can be tough in the beginning, but you will be amazed as the cravings slowly begin to disappear. As a former sugar addict, I know what you are thinking — "No way! I will still want that dessert." When you stick with the 10-day challenge, you begin to tune in to your body. Many times we use sugar to numb our feelings or to stop from feeling pain. We use sugar to deal with loneliness, boredom, stress or sadness. Tuning in to your body allows you to begin to feel these feelings. Sometimes this can be overwhelming, so it is important to get your support system set up. Especially with the added stress of infertility, a support person is crucial for your success.

> *It's all very simple. But maybe because it's so simple, it's also hard.*
> —Natuski Takaya

It seems like an easy solution: quit sugar. Sugar is everywhere, and you will have many temptations. Refer back to the intention that you set at the beginning of the book. When you are clear on your why, you can move mountains.

What You Need to Know

- Sugar is eight times more addictive than cocaine.
- Four grams of sugar equals 1 teaspoon of sugar. Read your labels or, better yet, don't buy anything in a box.

- Sugar creates a hormonal imbalance for both men and women.
- Sugar creates insulin resistance, and insulin resistance may prevent the body from ovulating.
- If you have candida, you will crave sugar, as sugar is fuel for candida.
- Get familiar with sugar alternatives such as maple syrup, brown rice syrup and stevia.

From Your Coach
What are your thoughts on sugar?
You can't give it up. You are defiantly addicted. You use it when you are bored, lonely and sad. It helps to numb your feelings. Sit with the thoughts for a few minutes. Grab your journal. Get curious with your thoughts. No judgment or guilt.

What may be holding you back from eliminating sugar?
Fear that you will give up one of your life's pleasure (you can still have the brownie and ice cream, but now it will be processed sugar free). You may have doubt that you can even give it up. Your cravings are very strong. You may even feel overwhelmed by all the decisions that need to be made. Remember, these thoughts and emotions are completely normal.

What is one step you can take today to eliminate sugar from your diet?
Substitute sugar in your coffee or tea with stevia, or swap your cookie habit for an apple. Commit to one step today.

Who will be your support?
Partner, friend or coach.

Visualize how you will feel when you eliminate sugar from your diet.
Envision feeling peaceful, calm with no cravings

What Is Next?
Could your daily cracker and bread habit have an impact on your fertility? Is gluten-free a fad, or could you really have a food intolerance or allergy?

Handy Resources
"Is Sugar Toxic?" *New York Times*
   http://www.nytimes.com/2011/04/17/magazine/mag-17Sugar-t.html?pagewanted=all&_r=0
   Glycemic index and load for 100+ foods
   http://www.health.harvard.edu/newsweek/Glycemic_index_and_glycemic_load_for_100_foods.htm
   Learn how to treat type 1 and type 2 diabetes, gestational diabetes with nutrition.
   http://www.drfuhrman.com/disease/Diabetes.aspx

References
1. *http://www.sciencedirect.com/science/article/pii/S0015028202032478*
3. *articles.mercola.com/sites/articles/archive/2007/08/23/is-sugar-moreaddictive-than-cocaine.aspx*
4. *http://www.womenshealth.gov/publications/our-publications/fact-sheet/polycystic-ovary-syndrome.html*
5.*http://www.heart.org/HEARTORG/GettingHealthy/NutritionCenter/HealthyEating/Sugar-101_UCM_306024_Article.jsp*
6. *http://www.cbc.ca/fifth/episodes/2013-2014/the-secrets-of-sugar*
[7]. Ingalls, Lindsay. "The effects of brown rice syrup on blood sugar." *Livestrong.* N.p., 20 Jun 2011. Web. 22 Dec 2011.

<http://www.livestrong.com/article/474520-the-effects-of-brown-rice-syrup-on-blood-sugar/>.

8. "Maple Syrup." *World's Healthiest Foods*. N.p., n.d. Web. 22 Dec 2011. *<http://www.whfoods.com/genpage. php?tname=foodspice&dbid=115>*.

9. O'Connor, Anahad. "Can Eating Local Honey Cure Allergies." *NY Times*. N.p., 09 May 2011. Web. 1 Feb 2012. *<http://www.nytimes. com/2011/05/10/health/10really.html?_r=1>*.

10. Institute of Integrative Nutrition, Natural Sweeteners, 2012

11. O'Connor, Anahad. "Can Eating Local Honey Cure Allergies." *NY Times*. N.p., 09 May 2011. Web. 1 Feb 2012. *<http://www.nytimes. com/2011/05/10/health/10really.html?_r=1>*.

12. Institute for Integrative Nutrition, Healthy Snacks, 2012.

Ten

GLUTEN-FREE AND SIMPLE CARBOHYDRATES

We have figured out that sugar is toxic and impacts fertility. What about gluten? The current gluten-free craze sweeping the nation can be misleading, because not everyone is sensitive to gluten. However, for many of my clients, eliminating gluten transformed their health. Those breads, cakes and muffins can taste delicious, but for someone who is intolerant to gluten, it can cause a myriad of health problems such as bloating, gas, diarrhea, vomiting and migraine headaches.

Gluten is present in cereal grains such as barley, rye and wheat, and is responsible for the elastic texture of dough. Gluten is what gives the final product its chewy texture. Gluten is also used as a food additive in the form of a flavouring, stabilizing or thickening agent, often hidden under "maltodextrin," "dextrine," and "dextrose." So watch out for it when you are shopping, as it may be in products that you do not expect. Some people that are gluten intolerant can still tolerate the ancient grains such as kamut and spelt. Although kamut and spelt still contain gluten, they are typically not as highly processed as white or whole wheat flour. It is important to still exercise caution, as you may experience a reaction. For anyone with celiac disease, gluten must be avoided.

Celiac Disease

Celiac disease is an autoimmune disease that damages the villi of the small intestine and interferes with absorption of nutrients from food. Approximately 1% of the population has celiac disease.[6] In order to be tested for celiac disease, you need to have gluten in your system to conduct the testing, so you may want to get tested before you eliminate gluten. However, you can still test negative for celiac disease and experience the symptoms of gluten intolerance.

Celiac disease can impact fertility and increase the risk of miscarriage. It may be the cause of up to 8% of unexplained infertility.[2] "Undiagnosed celiac disease can also create irregular menstrual cycles often associated with anovulation, and can cause amenorrhea (no menstruation) in up to 39% of women with undiagnosed celiac disease. All of these factors decrease fertility rates."[1] A study found that 2.5% of women suffering with endometriosis actually have undiagnosed celiac disease.[3] As well, there is an increased risk of miscarriage that occurs in 31% or more of undiagnosed celiac disease patients.[4] Celiac disease can also interfere with sperm production. Getting tested for celiac disease or eliminating gluten for three months is a good place to start as you begin to boost your fertility. You may not need to permanently eliminate gluten from your diet, but try it for at least three months, and it may improve your fertility.

Other Health Problems

Gluten can cause many health problems. Here are few that will benefit from an elimination of gluten: infertility, digestive upset, brain fog, diarrhea, constipation, joint pain, rashes, depression, anxiety, lupus, rheumatoid arthritis, hypothyroidism, acne and asthma.

If you suffer from any of the symptoms listed above — as well as digestive issues, PCOS and endometriosis — it is best to eliminate gluten for three months. Also, if you have a personal or family history of autoimmune disease, a gluten-free diet is recommended for three months, and if your symptoms improve, stay on the restricted diet. Women with PCOS may particularly benefit from a gluten-free diet, as many of the gluten-free grains such as quinoa, amaranth and brown rice are low on the glycemic index and will not spike blood sugar.

Eliminating Gluten

According to the National Foundation for Celiac Awareness, the good news is if you do have celiac disease or are gluten intolerant, the majority of women return to normal fertility rates for their age. Speak with your healthcare practitioner to determine when you can start trying to conceive, as you will want to maximize your body's nutrition before conception.

You can eliminate gluten and then gradually introduce it back into your system to determine if you have sensitivity. The 10-day challenge will offer you delicious gluten-free meals. At the end of the challenge, you can reintroduce gluten or wait three months to reintroduce gluten. The choice is up to you. If you decide to reintroduce gluten, introduce only one food item such as whole wheat pasta (consume two or three times per day for three days). Journal any symptoms such as joint pain, diarrhea, constipation, brain fog, digestive upset and acne. It is important to wait three days, as many people experience a delayed reaction to gluten.

I find that when I have gluten, my seasonal allergies flare up, my sinuses become congested, my joints start to ache and I experience some skin rashes. Gluten flares up my son's asthma, my daughter's and husband's sinuses. Anyone that has candida will need to eliminate gluten and start to heal the gut. Once the gut is healed, you may be able to reintroduce gluten. I have been gluten-free for almost two years. In the beginning it can be difficult navigating the gluten-free landscape, but the health benefits far outweigh the initial confusion.

Something else to consider is that many gluten-free products have loads of sugar and are simply not good for you. Watch out for gluten-free muffins, cookies and cakes, as many are loaded with refined sugar. Everyone seems to be jumping on the bandwagon and using gluten as a powerful marketing tool. Be careful what you choose or you could just be eating gluten-free junk food. These foods increase our blood sugar and adversely impact our fertility. Also, we need to watch out for simple carbohydrates, as these impacts our fertility.

The Harvard Nurses' Health Study found that eating too many simple carbohydrates could lower your chances of getting pregnant.[7] Simple carbohydrates or fast carbs like white bread, potatoes or diet colas are bad for your blood sugar.

Slow carbohydrates or complex carbohydrates, on the other hand, are slowly digested. They keep energy levels stable and can improve your fertility[7]. Steadier blood sugar levels and insulin levels may improver fertility. The higher the glycemic load of the food or the faster the carbohydrate hits the bloods sugar, the higher risk of ovulatory infertility.[8] Slow carbs include brown rice, pasta and dark breads. The study indicated that eating whole grains, beans, fruits and vegetables may improve ovulatory fertility

Try these low-glycemic-load options such as gluten-free grains, quinoa, millet, buckwheat, amaranth and brown rice. I like these options for baking: brown rice flour, almond flour (good but can be expensive), tapioca flour, teff flour and quinoa flour. Gluten-free oatmeal, quinoa flakes, quinoa, brown rice and chia seeds all make great breakfast grains. Tamari is a gluten-free option for soy sauce or coconut aminos.

You are on the path to making change.

Change is hard at first, messy in the middle and gorgeous at the end.
—Robin Sharma

What You Need to Know

- About 1% of the population has celiac disease.
- Celiac disease is associated with increased risk of miscarriage and irregular menstrual cycles. It can interfere with sperm production and is associated with endometriosis.
- You may test negative for celiac disease but still exhibit some of the symptoms and be gluten intolerant.
- Recommendation is to try the 10-day challenge, and you can introduce gluten, or may want to eliminate it for three months to determine if fertility improves. The choice is yours.
- Avoid slow or simple carbohydrates such as white bread and flours. These raise the blood sugar and increase the risk of ovulatory infertility.

From Your Coach
What are your thoughts about gluten?
Do you think it is a fad or could it be negatively impacting your fertility? Do you think the food will taste like cardboard or could it actually be fresh and delicious? Time to get curious with your thoughts. Remember, no judgment; grab your journal and start to write.

What may be holding you back when you think of eliminating gluten from your diet?
Do you think you will need to give up the pasta, baked goods or desserts? Truth is there are numerous gluten-free options to explore. The 10-day challenge will be your guide. You may even feel overwhelmed by all the decisions that need to be made. Remember, these thoughts and emotions are completely normal.

What is one action step you can take to go gluten-free?
Try substituting your white or whole wheat pasta for quinoa or brown rice pasta. You will be surprised how good it tastes. Commit to one step today.

Who will be your support system?
Partner, friend or coach.

Visualize how your body will feel when you eliminate gluten and simple carbohydrates.
Envision feeling lighter, less bloated, relaxed, joyful and peaceful.

What Is Next?
Could your daily glass of milk, yogurt or your addiction to cheese impact your fertility?

Handy Resources
Wheat Belly by William Davis: This is the book that started the gluten-free craze.
http://www.wheatbellyblog.com/
Grain Brain by David Perlmutter: No, it's not all in your head. Gluten intolerance affects the brain.
http://www.drperlmutter.com/
Marks Daily Apple
http://www.marksdailyapple.com/
Elana's Pantry: Great resource for gluten-free recipes.
http://www.elanaspantry.com/
Against All Grains: Another great website for gluten-free recipes.
http://againstallgrain.com/

References
1. *http://www.celiaccentral.org/research-news/ Celiac-Disease-Research/134/vobid--2030/*

2. http://www.celiaccentral.org/research-news/
Celiac-Disease-Research/134/vobid--2030/
3. http://humrep.oxfordjournals.org/content/early/2011/08/11/hum-rep.der263.short
4. http://www.celiaccentral.org/research-news/
Celiac-Disease-Research/134/vobid--2030/
6. http://www.celiaccentral.org/celiac-disease/facts-and-figures/
7. http://www.cgribben.com/RTC/WELL/Articles_files/Fats%20
Carbs.pdf
8. http://www.nature.com/ejcn/journal/v63/n1/abs/1602904a.html
9. http://www.ima.org.il/FilesUpload/IMAJ/0/45/22775.pdf

Eleven

DAIRY AND SOY

Y̶ou now know how gluten impacts fertility. What about dairy and soy?

Dairy

For many people dairy is a toxic food. That may sound shocking, since we have been programed to drink milk from the time we were weaned from our mothers. You may have heard that humans are the only mammal in the animal kingdom that consumes milk from another animal after being weaned. Time to rethink our dairy consumption. Many people are intolerant to dairy, and this can cause a myriad of health conditions such as sinusitis, eczema and acne, just to name a few.

It then came as a surprise that the Harvard Nurses' Health Study found that women who consumed full-fat milk or dairy products improved their chances of becoming pregnant. Consuming one serving a day of a full fat dairy food, particularly milk, decreased the chance of having ovulatory infertility.[3] The research from the study found consumption of low-fat dairy products reduced the likelihood of becoming pregnant. Wait a minute; I bet you thought skim milk was a better option than whole milk. When low-fat or skim milk is prepared, the whole milk is spun at high speeds to separate the fat from the water. When the fat is skimmed off the whole milk, this fat includes male sex hormones, prolactin and insulin-like growth factor-1. These male sex hormones impede fertility in women. Prolactin, the hormone that suppresses breast milk, can suppress ovulation. That's why women don't usually get pregnant if they are breastfeeding. Watch out, though, as whole-fat milk is loaded with calories, and added weight can affect your fertility.

Dairy is also one of the top allergens, and many people benefit from eliminating dairy from their diet. The best idea is to figure out if you are intolerant to dairy by removing it from your diet and then rechallenging it later. During the 10-day challenge, you will not consume any dairy. You can eliminate dairy for three months, or if you wish to rechallenge dairy, introduce one dairy food such as whole milk (consume two or three times per day for three days). Journal any symptoms. Look for symptoms such as bloating, gas, digestive upset or sinus congestion. If you experience any symptoms, you know that you are intolerant. Intolerance to dairy affects both male and female fertility. The key is to heal the inflammation in your gut, since partially digested proteins get into your bloodstream. This may affect the ovaries and the testicles and their ability to function. When the food is removed, the gut can begin to heal and fertility can be restored.[8]

Many people underestimate the amount of dairy they consume. When I ask clients how much dairy they consume, the usual reply is, "I don't consume much." But when they think about it further, they realize they really do consume more than they think. Usually, it is in the form of cheese. In 1970 a person in America ate an average of 8 pounds of cheese per year. Now it is 23 pounds of cheese per year.[4] Consumption has almost tripled.

Another question I hear a lot is, "But where will I get my calcium?" The dairy board has done a great job of marketing the supposed benefits of milk. Those ads that have celebrities smiling with milk mustaches are very clever. It makes us believe that milk is essential for healthy bones and teeth and is the only option for calcium. Well, nothing could be further from the truth. Studies have shown that dairy consumption actually causes more osteoporosis and more porous bones, leading to fractures.[5] Cows and elephants eat only plant food and get ample calcium for their bones. If they can have strong bones without dairy, we can too.

"Drink your milk, it does a body good." Maybe it is time for us to look at the affects of dairy a little differently. If you determine that you are not intolerant to milk and still wish to consume it, be sure to drink organic milk that is hormone and antibiotic free.

Soy
Some people think that substituting soy for dairy is a healthy option. I know I did this for years, thinking I was making a healthy choice. Now there is evidence that soy harms the thyroid, contributes to breast cancer, is dangerous for babies and could contribute to erectile dysfunction and low sperm count.[7] *The American Journal of Clinical Nutrition* found that women who consumed 60 grams of soy protein experienced decreases in follicle-stimulating hormone and luteinizing hormone. Soy consumption could equal decreased fertility for women. Although some studies have shown improvement with menopausal symptoms such as hot flashes with soy consumption.[6]

Soy is also considered one of the top seven food allergens, along with gluten, dairy, eggs, corn, peanuts and sugar. If you are currently consuming soy on a daily basis and experiencing hormonal imbalance, ovulatory infertility, menstrual problems, erectile dysfunction, low sperm count, breast enlargement (men) and decreased libido, try eliminating if from your diet. Start with the 10-day challenge, and you can rechallenge soy. Start with one soy product such as tofu (consume two or three times per day for three days), and journal any symptoms such as abdominal pain, breast tenderness, sinus congestion, acne, brain fog and joint pain. If you experience any symptoms, you know that you are intolerant. You may simply want to eliminate it for three months and then rechallenge. If you are not consuming soy and are experiencing ovulatory infertility or hormonal imbalance, you may want to add it to your diet for three months.

Every body is different. There is not a one-size-fits-all approach to boosting fertility. Here are some recommendations to follow:

- Consume only one or two soy products per week. Soy naturally contains toxins, phytoestrogens and antinutrients. It's best to consume fermented soy products such as miso, tempeh and soybeans.
- Limit your consumption of processed soy (tofu, soy lunch meats, soy yogurt, soy burgers and soy cheese). These unfermented soy products cause a myriad of health problems such as higher risk of infertility, increased risk of breast cancer, hypothyroidism, just to name a few.
- Ensure you purchase nongenetically modified soy products. Soybeans are a highly genetically modified crop. Look for organic nongenetically modified soy.
- Soy is one of the top allergens, especially genetically modified soy. Many people think they are eating a healthy alternative to dairy, but the symptoms of a soy allergy can include abdominal pain, diarrhea, nausea, sinus congestion and skin rashes.
- Try some of these delicious nondairy milks. Everyone has their favourite, so feel free to try some different options!
  - Unsweetened almond milk: Creamy, just a little sweet and high in vitamin E. Blue Diamond Almond Breeze is my favourite. I toss it in smoothies, drink it by itself and bake with it.
  - Unsweetened hemp milk: Rich in Omega-3s, its delicious, but won't get you high!
  - Unsweetened coconut milk: It's creamy and delicious.

Use it in baking, smoothies or for ice cream. Try So Delicious Coconut Milk.

- Unsweetened rice milk: Rice milk is thinner in consistency. Try Rice Dream Enriched Original.

There is a difference between interest and commitment. When you're interested in something, you do it only when it's convenient. When you're committed to something, you accept no excuses, only results.
—Kenneth H. Blanchard

Dairy can be difficult for many people to eliminate. Some of my clients tell me that they never knew they were feeling so bad until they feel so great.

Are you committed? Refer back to your intention.

What You Need to Know

- Dairy is a toxic food and is one of the top food allergens.
- The Harvard Nurses' Health Study found that whole milk increased fertility, while skim milk decreased fertility.
- Soy intake may contribute to ovulatory infertility, low sperm count and erectile dysfunction.
- Try the 10-day challenge first, and eliminate dairy

and soy from your diet. Rechallenge and note any
side affects.
- If you decide to drink dairy, drink organic milk that
is hormone and antibiotic free.

From Your Coach
What are you thoughts on dairy and soy?
Dairy is supposed to be good for me. I've been taught that all my
life. Could it really be affecting my fertility? Time to get curious
with your thoughts. Remember, no judgment; grab your journal
and start to write.

What may be holding you back from eliminating dairy and soy?
What will you put in your cereal? What about your love of cheese?
You love your soy milk, so how will you give it up? You may feel
overwhelmed by all the decisions that need to be made. Remember,
these thoughts and emotions are completely normal.

What is one action step that you can take to eliminate dairy and soy?
You can substitute almond milk in your morning cereal, or you can try
coconut milk in your morning smoothie. Commit to one step today.

Who will be your support?
Partner, friend or coach.

Visualize how your body will feel without dairy and soy.
Envision feeling lighter, less congested, with clearer skin and a
smooth digestion.

What Is Next?
We have been taught for so long to avoid fat at all costs. What if this
well-meaning advice was all wrong? Does fat impact your fertility?

Handy Resources
Check out this movie — *Got the Facts About Milk?*
http://www.milkdocumentary.com/
Learn more from T. Colin Campbell Foundation on why we don't need milk.
http://nutritionstudies.org/no-body-needs-milk/
Listen up men! Dairy consumption is directly related to prostate cancer.
http://www.pcrm.org/health/cancer-resources/diet-cancer/type/prostate-cancer
The dangers of soy and the effects of soy on health
http://articles.mercola.com/sites/articles/archive/2010/12/04/soy-dangers-summarized.aspx
http://archive.ahrq.gov/clinic/epcsums/soysum.htm

References
1. *http://www.ima.org.il/FilesUpload/IMAJ/0/45/22775.pdf*
2. *http://www.sciencedirect.com/science/article/pii/S089990071000359X*
3. http://humrep.oxfordjournals.org/content/22/5/1340.short
4. *http://grist.org/list/we-eat-three-times-as-much-cheese-now-as-we-did-in-1970/*
5. *http://pcrm.org/media/commentary/dairy-products-and-bone-health*
6. *http://archive.ahrq.gov/clinic/epcsums/soysum.htm*
7. *http://humrep.oxfordjournals.org/content/23/11/2584.short*
8. *https://www.foodintol.com/have-a-healthy-pregnancy*

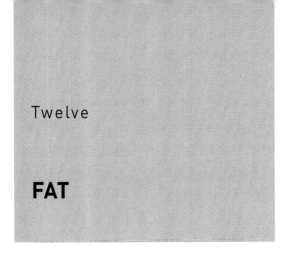

Twelve

FAT

We know how dairy and soy can impact fertility, and it is now time to turn our attention to fat. Most people have been taught that all fats are bad for our health. Turns out that some fats are good for our fertility, and some fats are not so good.

There are four different types of fats: saturated, monounsaturated, polyunsaturated and trans fats. The first three fats should be included in your diet, and trans fat should be eliminated. The Harvard Nurses' Health Study found that trans fats threaten ovulation and conception, as well as harm the heart and blood vessels. Let's run down the different types of fats.

Monounsaturated Fats
These fats are good at lowering cholesterol and the body's sensitivity to insulin and inflammation. Be careful, as these oils are unstable at high temperatures and have the potential to convert to trans fatty acids. For high heat, coconut oil is the best, and for lower temperatures, cold pressed olive oil is preferred.

Good sources include olives, olive oils, hazelnuts, almonds, cashews, nut butters, avocados, sesame seeds and pumpkin seeds.

Polyunsaturated Fats
These fats contain omega-3 fatty acids and omega-6 fatty acids. Omega-6 is inflammatory to the body, and omega-3 is anti-inflammatory. Our body needs both, and, ideally, we should be consuming

at a 2:1 ratio. These fats are good for fertility. (See more information under "Essential Fatty Acids" following.)

Good sources include legumes, walnuts, chia seeds, hemp seeds, sesame seeds and fatty fish such as tuna, salmon, herring and anchovies.

Saturated Fats

These should be used infrequently. They raise cholesterol and increase risk for a stroke or heart disease. They are found in high-fat meats, whole milk and tropical oils such as palm oil, palm kernel oil and coconut oil. However, tropical oils can be used in moderation and do not contain cholesterol.

Good sources include coconut oil and palm oil.

Trans Fats

These are to be avoided. The Harvard Nurses' Health Study found that trans fats increased inflammation throughout the body, which interferes with ovulation, conception and early embryonic development. Obtaining just 2% of total calories from trans fats instead of healthier monounsaturated fats was associated with a doubled risk for this type of infertility. In addition, each 2% increase in trans fat consumption as a replacement for carbohydrates brought a 73% greater risk of ovulation-related infertility, after adjusting for other known and suspected infertility risk factors, according to the study.[4] Trans fats also increase the risk of miscarriage.[2] Read labels, and watch out for partially hydrogenated vegetable oil or vegetable shortening, as these are trans fats. Better yet, don't eat anything from a box.

Canada has not banned trans fats as other countries such as Denmark, Iceland and Switzerland have. Canada limits the trans fats in margarines and vegetables oils to 2%, and 5% of the fat content for foods such as cookies, pastries, frozen desserts and puddings. Since 1975, government, advertisers, doctors and nutrition experts have advocated a diet low in fat. What this fad has failed to address is the difference between low-quality saturated fats contained in junk foods and mostly animal products and naturally occurring unsaturated fats found mostly in plants.[5]

We have been taught for many years that low-fat, no-fat, calorie-free foods are the way to lose weight. These products are manufactured with added sugar, salt and additives. They need to add these products so the food will actually taste good. The sugar is especially dangerous because chronic consumption of sugar dulls the brains mechanism to feel full. When we eat these "fat-free" products, we inadvertently set ourselves up to always feel hungry and unsatisfied. There is nothing in these products that makes us satisfied. The brain doesn't get the message to stop eating. This is a huge revelation to anyone trying to lose weight. Your inability to lose weight is not your fault. It's the fructose that is added to all the products that keep you feeling hungry and has caused the current obesity epidemic.

Fat Is Not the Enemy
Good fats from monounsaturated and polyunsaturated fats improve your chances of getting pregnant. Human beings actually need lots of high-quality fat in our diets. Here are some reasons why:

- for the production of hormones
- to protect internal organs and protect them from cold
- to burn energy when carbs are scarce
- to cover every single body and brain cell
- to make hair and skin lustrous
- to keep sex drive from waning
- to maintain mental stability and concentration
- to prevent carbohydrate cravings
- to keep bowels regular

Since many of us are eating processed foods, we are deficient in healthy fats.

The body can't produce these fats on its own; you must get them through food.

Essential Fatty Acids

As mentioned previously, polyunsaturated fats can be broken down into two categories: omega-3 and omega-6. They are both essential fatty acids.

Omega-3s

These have powerful anti-inflammatory properties and are essential for normal fetal growth and development.[7] Omega-3 fatty acid levels have also been associated with decreased breast cancer risk.[6]

Good food sources include:

- unrefined flax oil, walnut oil, pumpkin seed oil
- hemp seeds
- avocados
- dark leafy greens (kale, spinach, purslane, mustard greens, collards)
- sesame seeds, chia seeds, flax seeds
- cold pressed unrefined canola oil
- Brazil nuts
- salmon, mackerel, sardines, albacore tuna

Omega-6s

These cause inflammation, but are still needed for the body to properly function. The standard Western diet is high in omega-6s, and many people are eating a ratio of 15:1 omega-6s to omega-3s, when a ratio of 2:1 is recommended.

Good food sources include:

- flaxseed oil, flaxseeds, flaxseed meal
- hemp seed oil, hemp seeds
- grapeseed oil
- pumpkin seeds, pine nuts, pistachio nuts, sunflower seeds (raw)
- olive oil, olives
- borage oil, evening primrose oil, black currant seed oil, chestnut oil
- chicken

Drizzle oils on your salads (you'll wonder why you ever ate the store-bought salad dressing) and on your vegetables. If you have a hard time digesting nuts, soak them overnight to activate the sprouting process. You can strain and dry them and either roast or eat them raw. Chewing the nut well will also help with digestion.

Best oils for cooking are:

- coconut Oil (Great for weight loss, as the body quickly converts it to energy.)
- extra virgin olive oil
- sesame oil

Symptoms Caused by Deficiencies in Essential Fatty Acids[2-4]

- abnormalities in the liver and the kidneys
- reduced growth rates
- decreased immune function

- depression
- dryness of the skin

Benefits of Adequate Consumption of Essential Fatty Acids[2-4]

- prevention of atherosclerosis
- reduced incidence of heart disease and stroke
- relief from symptoms of ulcerative colitis, menstrual pain and joint pain

Now its time to break the bad habits and make better ones. Be kind to yourself along the journey. Recognize that what you are doing for your health. Not many people have the courage or discipline do to. As you discover how your fertility can be impacted by food, take small steps every day. Start to walk the talk. And remember not to preach; actions speak louder than words.

What You Need to Know

- Avoid trans fats, as they increase your risk of ovulatory infertility and miscarriage.
- Add monounsaturated and polyunsaturated fats such as omega-3s and omega-6s to your diet.

From Your Coach
What are you thoughts about fats and trans fat?
How will I eliminate trans fat from my diet? Could it really be affecting my fertility? Time to get curious with your thoughts. Remember, no judgment; grab your journal and start to write.

What may be holding you back from adding healthy fats to your diet?

How will I incorporate fat into my diet? I thought fat was bad for me. I'm not sure if I even like the good fats. You may even feel overwhelmed by all the decisions that need to be made. Remember, these thoughts and emotions are completely normal.

What is one step you can take to eliminate trans fats from your diet?

Switch up your morning breakfast routine, and start with one of the 10-day challenge smoothies. Commit to one step today.

Who will support you?

Partner, friend or coach.

Visualize how your body will feel when you are eating healthy fats.

Envision feeling energized, satisfied, with no cravings.

What Is Next?

Could your daily glass of wine or beer be affecting your fertility?

Handy Resources

Time to end the low-fat myth.

http://www.hsph.harvard.edu/nutritionsource/ what-should-you-eat/fats-and-cholesterol/

References

1. *http://ajcn.nutrition.org/content/85/1/231.short*
2. *http://www.sciencedirect.com/science/article/pii/ S0015028207013805*

3. *http://www.sciencedirect.com/science/article/pii/S0753332202002536 - delete #3*

4. *http://www.webmd.com/infertility-and-reproduction/news/20070112/trans-fats-infertility*

5. Integrative Nutrition, Joshua Rosenthal, 2013

6. *http://www.pcrm.org/health/health-topics/essential-fatty-acids*

7. *http://www.pnas.org/content/88/11/4835.short*

Thirteen

ALCOHOL

We learned about avoiding trans fats and adding healthy fats to our meals. Now its time to talk about what we drink. Many of us already know about the warnings of excess alcohol consumption during pregnancy. What we may not know is how alcohol consumption affects our ability to get pregnant.

The Harvard Nurses' Study concluded that moderate drinking, up to one drink per day, did not affect fertility[1] That news may seems shocking, but don't bring out the vodka and tonic just yet. One study of nearly 5,000 women with infertility due to endometriosis showed that endometriosis was 50% higher in women who consumed even moderate amounts of alcohol (up to one drink per day) compared to those who didn't.[3] Another study of more than 29,000 men revealed that alcohol consumption was a risk factor for lower semen volume.[1] Yet another study revealed that consumption of as few as four alcoholic drinks per week is associated with a decrease in IVF live birth rates.[2]

So, there is some food for thought. Although there seems to be some conflicting reports, it is always better to err on the side of caution. Forgoing alcohol when you are trying to conceive is always recommended.

Numerous studies support that heavy drinking while pregnant can harm the fetus and lead to fetal alcohol syndrome and other cognitive impairments to the unborn child.

For some people, giving up alcohol may seem impossible. For many people, alcohol is linked to relaxation. Having a drink after a hard day, celebrating an occasion or getting together with friends for a drink — it's fun!

Alcohol consumption is part of our culture, and there is pressure to conform. Key is to bring awareness to your habits around drinking. Does the drink signal relaxation? Do you use it as a reward? Such as having a drink after a challenging work week? Do you use alcohol for social situations? Many people use alcohol to numb themselves and stop from feeling their emotions. Time to get curious about your thoughts and actions.

When you begin to eliminate alcohol from your diet, remember the crowding-out principle. Have a glass of water before each drink and you will be less likely to drink as much. Be kind to yourself. Alcohol is full of sugar, and we know that sugar is eight times more addictive than cocaine. That's why alcohol can be so difficult to quit. Check to make sure you are eating enough protein. This will reduce your cravings.

If the 10-day challenge overlaps with a special occasion, you can add sparking water to the wine so you can enjoy yourself. If you happen to slip up, remember, you don't need to give up. Just start again the next day.

This book does not deal with serious addiction. If you think you may have a problem with alcohol, please consult your physician. The link to Alcoholics Anonymous is listed for your reference.

The path to wellness can have many bumps. Rewards are crucial to keep you on track. When I ask my clients how they reward themselves, many have never even considered giving themselves a reward. Buy yourself some flowers; spend time by yourself with a good book; book a massage; throw on some loud music, and dance around the house; treat yourself to a meal at a restaurant (vegan, of course); or watch your favourite guilty pleasure on TV. When you give yourself a reward, you'll be more apt to stick with the program.

What You Need to Know

- The Harvard Nurses' Health Study found that moderate drinking (up to one drink per day) did not affect fertility.
- Other studies found that alcohol consumption was a factor in low semen production and endometriosis.
- Use the crowding-out principle[4], and drink a glass of water before your alcoholic beverage, or dilute your drink with water.

From Your Coach
What are your thoughts about eliminating alcohol from your diet?
You don't know how you will cope. You reward yourself with alcohol after a stressful day. You use it to celebrate. You like how it tastes with your meal. However, you now know that it could be impacting your fertility. Time to get curious with your thoughts. Remember, no judgment; grab your journal and start to write.

What is holding you back from eliminating alcohol from your diet?
How do you deal with your difficult emotions? Do you numb them with alcohol? Time to sit with your feelings and journal how you feel. Reach out for help if the emotions are too painful. You may even feel overwhelmed by all the decisions that need to be made. Remember, these thoughts and emotions are completely normal.

What is one step you can take today to eliminate alcohol from your diet?
Remember the crowding-out principle. Drink a glass of water before you have alcohol, or add water to your alcoholic drink. Commit to one step today.

Who can be your support system as you eliminate alcohol?
Partner, friend, coach or therapist.

What Is Next?
What is the best drink of choice for boosting fertility?

Handy Resources
Here is the website for Alcoholics Anonymous.
   http://www.aa.org

References
1. *http://books.google.ca/books?hl=en&lr=&id=rZs6Aw
AAQBAJ&oi=fnd&pg=PA84&dq=ALCOHOL+AND+FE
RTILITY&ots=rOF-fA_QW6&sig=9Jv_OJlE_akVdEpY-
wp_K36Flw5M#v=onepage&q=ALCOHOL%20AND%20
FERTILITY&f=false*
2. *http://journals.lww.com/greenjournal/Abstract/2011/01000/
Effect_of_Alcohol_Consumption_on_In_Vitro.20.aspx*
3. *http://ajph.aphapublications.org/doi/abs/10.2105/AJPH.84.9.1429*
4. Institute for Integrative Nutrition, Crowding Out, 2012

Fourteen

WATER

We know that alcohol can adversely affect your ability to conceive. How about a different drink of choice? Cool, refreshing water. Some 70% of our body is made up of water. Keeping hydrated is good for reproductive health and for your body both preconception and during pregnancy. Water lubricates and cushions your tissues and organs.

Blood flow and proper oxygenation are crucial for healthy ovaries and eggs. Dehydration causes the blood to become thick and decreases circulation in the body. This decreases blood flow to the ovaries. Water also aids in production of cervical mucus. This is needed for the sperm to get to the egg. Water helps to detoxify the body. Time to start drinking your water.

Aim for eight glasses of water daily. Or a good rule of thumb is to divide your weight in half, and that's how many ounces of water you should drink per day. For example, 120 pounds — 60 fluid ounces — or 7.5 cups. Exact water requirements vary widely among individuals. Listen to your body and learn how much works for you.

Many of us are chronically dehydrated. We never stop to take the time to drink enough water. When we eat the standard Western diet, which is high in flour products (crackers, cookies, breads), water consumption is even more important. When we eat a lot of dried flour products, we require more water in our system to counteract the drying effect of the flour. When we add more vegetables into the diet, our need to drink water diminishes, as we are getting sufficient water from salads, soups and veggies drinks, just to name a few. It's best to drink the water before your meal, but if you have a small drink during your meal, that's OK too.

If the taste of pure water really doesn't appeal to you, try adding one of the following to jazz it up:

- lemon and lime slices (Add some mint for extra flavour.)
- strawberry and basil
- cucumbers
- apple with cinnamon stick

These infusions are for when you get sick of water, so save these for a special treat. The more water you drink, the more you will begin to crave water. Get used to drinking one or two glasses of water when you wake up in the morning.

Many people get hung up on the type of water to drink: bottled, reverse osmosis, carbon filtered. It is important to remember to drink water instead of pop, coffee, tea, juice or alcohol.

Once you are in the habit of drinking water, here are few tips to consider. The best option is to drink spring water or filtered water. Reverse osmosis is the preferred option, but it can be costly. Grab a filter for your tap such as a Brita. Avoid bottled water if possible. Harmful chemicals from the plastic can leach into the water, and the excess bottles harm the environment. Tap water is convenient but may not always be the safest option, depending on your city's purification system.

What You Need to Know

- Dehydration can decrease circulation in the body and decrease blood flow to the ovaries.
- Divide your weight in half to determine how many

ounces of water to drink. For example, 120 pounds —
60 fluid ounces — or 7.5 cups.

- Try some water infuser recipes to jazz up your water.
- Choose filtered water. Reverse osmosis is preferred.
- Don't drink water from plastic bottles.

From Your Coach
What are your thoughts to adding water to your daily regime?
You wonder how you will have time to drink so much water. Does
the body really need so much water? I don't feel dehydrated. I've
never really liked water. Time to get curious with your thoughts.
Remember, no judgment; grab your journal and start to write.

What is holding you back from drinking water every day?
Concerned about going to the bathroom every minute as your body
gets adjusted to the increased fluids? You will go a little more, but after a while you body will absorb the water more effectively. Don't like
the taste of water? Add one of the water infuser recipes to your glass.
You may feel overwhelmed by all the decisions that need to be made.
Remember, these thoughts and emotions are completely normal.

What is one step you can take to add water to your diet?
Purchase a stainless steel or glass water container. Drink two glasses of water when you wake up. Commit to one step today.

Who will support you?
Partner, friend or coach.

*Visualize fueling your body with the hydrating and beneficial
affects of water.*
Envision feeling energized, having a smoother digestion and feeling
more rested, calm, light and peaceful.

113

What Is Next?
You know you need to exercise daily, but could your daily exercise program affect your fertility?

Handy Resources
Fruit infuser recipes to add to your water
   http://www.loseweightbyeating.com/category/zero-calorie-drinks/
   The risk of water fluoridation
   http://cof-cof.ca/faqs/

Fifteen

MOVEMENT

We learned the importance of hydration to supercharge your fertility. Now, let's figure out how movement factors into your fertility. Exercise is definitely good for fertility, but the key is to not overdo it. If you currently don't exercise, it's time to strap on your running shoes. If you exercise regularly, it's time to pick up the intensity. But it's important not too exercise too vigorously, as too much exercise can interfere with ovulation. [1]

Moderate exercise is recommended to increase fertility; however, extreme exercise is associated with decreased ability to conceive or with luteal phase defect.[2] Athletes of any kind have a higher rates of amenorrhea (cessation of period) than the general population.[3] Regular exercise before IVF may negatively affect outcomes. One study showed that women who exercised four or more hours per week predicted an IVF cycle that was 50% less effective. Cardiovascular exercise was shown to be the most detrimental, with a 30% lower chance of successful pregnancy after first IVF cycle.[4]

Male fertility is less impacted by exercise. Although, if a man is participating in extreme exercise and is experiencing fertility problems, it may be a good idea to exercise at a moderate level.[4]

OK, we all know we need to move more. We get it. Exercise is good for you. Here are some of the benefits.[6]

- Exercise helps you to control your weight.
- Exercise helps combat health problems such as heart

disease, diabetes and arthritis.

- Exercise improves your mood by stimulating brain chemical to help you feel more relaxed, and it can improve your self-confidence and sleep.
- Exercise boosts your energy by delivering oxygen to your system. It also helps your cardiovascular system work more efficiently.
- Exercise revs up your sex life (you look and feel better). Regular physical activity leads to enhanced arousal for woman. Men who exercise regularly are less likely to have problems with erectile dysfunction.

The daily recommended dose of movement is 30 minutes. It doesn't matter how you incorporate the 30 minutes into your day. If you are pressed for time, try 10 minutes three times per day. For many of my clients, when they get stressed or busy, the first thing to go is the exercise routine. Funny how it's the thing that is most needed to combat stress. It releases endorphins and gives you that natural high. Walking is the easiest and cheapest form of exercise. All you need is a pair of running shoes and a sidewalk — a walking buddy helps too.

Need some more motivation? Try a fitness tracker. It's a bracelet that tracks your movement, sleep and nutrition. This goes a few steps further than the pedometer. The app displays your data, lets you add things like meals and mood and delivers insights that keep you moving forward. You can download the information to your mobile device and check out your statistics. Gyms are starting to get on the bandwagon too. Your personal trainer can access your statistics while you are away from the gym and determine just how "good" you have been keeping up with the recommendations. It's your very own personal virtual coach!

Take this survey to find out what exercise is best for your body, mind and spirit.

http://the8colorsoffitness.com/

When you discover your fitness preference, you can create an exercise program that you will never quit. Include some of the following in your exercise routine: some cardio (brisk walking, biking, swimming or dancing); strength training (lifting weights or using resistance bands); stretching (yoga or Pilates).

Don't like to leave your house? Do you like working out in the comfort of your own home? Does going to the gym fill you with dread? Here's your solution. Work out in the comfort of your own home with your own personal trainer. Check out the new crop of online live workout classes. It's similar to doing workout DVDs with one big difference — the instructor can see you and offer valuable feedback during the workout. All you need is a webcam.

Bottom line: Pull back on the vigorous exercise. If you don't exercise, start today, as it will help you lose weight and enhance your fertility.

Before you begin a new exercise program ensure you speak with your physician or healthcare practitioner.

Do it now; some time later becomes never. There will always be a reason why you can't start a new habit. — too busy, too something. When you take small steps every day, you start to notice results. Maybe you start with placing your running shoes by the door when you come home from work. You commit to going for a five-minute walk. If you are addicted to vigorous exercise, commit to the same five-minute walk, but slow down. Really notice your surroundings. Inhale the fresh air. Smalls steps each day amount to huge success.

What You Need to Know

- Exercise is good for fertility.
- Too much vigorous exercise may impede your fertility.
- Too much exercise before IVF may reduce your chances of conception.
- Take the survey to discover what type of exercise routine you prefer.
- For maximum fertility, if you don't exercise, start today. However, make sure you pull back on vigorous exercise.

From Your Coach
What are you thoughts around exercise?
You could never add exercise to your day. You are way too busy. What will everyone think when you start walking? They may stare at you, and you will feel uncomfortable. You need the vigorous exercise; it's how you unwind. But how can you pull back? Could exercise affect your fertility? Time to get curious with your thoughts. Remember, no judgment; grab your journal and start to write.

What is holding you back from incorporating exercise or pulling back from a more vigorous exercise routine?
You are addicted to vigorous exercise. You need it to get through your day. The thought of exercise makes you want to jump on the coach and stay there all day. You may feel overwhelmed by all the decisions that need to be made. Remember, these thoughts and emotions are completely normal.

What is one step you can take today to add or pull back on your exercise routine?
You will walk for five minutes today. You will buy a new pair of running shoes. You will get an exercise buddy. Commit to one step today.

Who will be your support?
Partner, friend or coach.

Visualize yourself exercising.
Envision yourself feeling strong, flexible and invigorated.

What Is Next?
How does your weight affect your ability to conceive?

Handy Resources
Article on which fitness tracker may be right for you
http://well.blogs.nytimes.com/projects/activity-trackers#jawbone-up
Virtual trainer sites
www.powhow.com
www.wello.com
www.balletbeautiful.com
www.bodsforbroads.com

References
1. *http://journals.lww.com/epidem/Abstract/2002/03000/Physical_Activity,_Body_Mass_Index,_and_Ovulatory.13.aspx*
2. *http://europepmc.org/abstract/MED/12972877*
3. *http://link.springer.com/chapter/10.1007/978-3-642-70743-8_9#page-1*

4. *http://journals.lww.com/greenjournal/abstract/2006/10000/effects_of_lifetime_exercise_on_the_outcome_of_in.18.aspx*
5. *http://link.springer.com/article/10.2165/00007256-199315030-00002#page-1*
6. *http://www.mayoclinic.org/healthy-living/fitness/in-depth/exercise/art-20048389?pg=2*
7. *http://www.besthealthmag.ca/get-healthy/fitness/fitness-trend-webcam-classes*

Sixteen

WEIGHT

We figured out how movement can affect your fertility. Now, its time to talk about weight. This can be a touchy subject. Our society is obsessed with everything "skinny." However, there has been a backlash against the unachievable skinny role model, and we are now seeing more average-sized people in the media. This is still the exception and not the rule. Since we all come in different shapes and sizes, my philosophy as a health coach is not to count calories, but to allow my clients to tune in to how their body feels when they eat. Many times we are on automatic pilot and don't even realize we are stuffing food into our mouth — when we aren't even hungry! It could be the stress of trying to conceive, catching up on your ever-mounting to-do list or trying to be everything to everyone. When we tune in to what we really need such as time for ourselves, a hug or a true connection with our partner or loved one, the weight starts to melt off.

The statistics don't lie; moderate weight loss does impact fertility. If you are struggling with ovulatory infertility, according to one study, losing 5% to 10% of your current weight is often enough to improve ovulation.[3] This is especially helpful for women with PCOS, as weight loss can help to restore menstruation and ovulation.[2]

The Harvard Nurses' Health Study found that women considered obese — with a body mass index (BMI) above 30 — had an increased risk of ovulatory infertility. Women considered overweight —

with a BMI between 25 and 29.9 — also had an increased risk of ovulatory infertility.[1]

Excess weight can also affect men's ability to conceive. One study suggested that overweight and obese men are more likely than their normal-weight peers to produce lower numbers of sperm counts or no sperm at all.[4]

Underweight women, with a BMI below 19, have an increased risk of miscarriage.[5] Low BMI also affects men and is associated with lower sperm counts.

Now, all of this can be overwhelming when you are trying to conceive. It's not about going on a restrictive crash diet and depriving yourself of all enjoyable foods. If you are underweight, it's about trying to figure out how to eat the proper nutrients to gain weight. We are surrounded with toxic foods, and they are addictive. It's not your fault. The food industry has done a great job of marketing. Approximately one in four Canadians and one in three Americans are obese. Many of us already know these statistics, but we are so addicted to the toxic food that we can't stop eating it.

Once we set an intention and take small steps every day, we start to see results.

I know it can be scary. During the 10-day challenge, you'll give up meat (if you have candida, you will may still need to keep animal protein), dairy, gluten, processed sugar, caffeine and alcohol. First question is how will you give up your steak, cheese, bread and sugary sweets. Too much meat increases ovulatory infertility. Dairy and gluten are two of the top food triggers that cause food intolerance and sensitivity in many people. Sugar is highly addictive, and the food industry has done a good job of hiding it in many supposedly healthy foods. These toxic foods cause cravings and keep us unsatisfied and constantly hungry.

After the toxic foods leave your system, you will have a renewed sense of energy, and you will no longer be held hostage by your cravings.

If after the 10-day challenge you require more support, my one-on-one coaching programs offer individual support to guide you through the program. I keep you on track and remind you of your intention. As your guide by the side, I hold you accountable. The idea is not to criticize you if don't meet one of your goals, but together we figure out what got in your way and get you back on the track.

In the hustle and bustle of daily living, many of us forget to truly sit down and savour our food. We stop at the drive-thru, rush home and start working on our to-do list. When you are preparing your body for conception, it is especially important to slow down. Learn to say no. You can't do it all. And you know what? You don't have to.

Eating Mindfully
Here are some tips to eat mindfully.

It is best to eat with no distractions: Yes, that means turning off the TV, putting down the book or magazine. It's time to keep your meal times calm and relaxing.

Give thanks for the meal: It is an especially good idea to thank the cook; she or he will be more apt to cook again for you when you express your thanks.

Take your time to chew each bite: Learn to savour your food instead of stuffing it into your mouth. Macrobiotics has a brown rice fast where you eat nothing but brown rice for ten days and you chew each bite 100 times. Sound a little extreme? During my time at the Kushi Institute in Beckett, Massachusetts, when I was studying macrobiotics, I was really able to start to chew my food. I started to take smaller portions in my mouth and then chew each bite. It was like I could feel the nutrients fueling my body. For the first time I was able to slow down and really enjoy my food. And you know what? I was actually satisfied for longer.

Eat only when you are hungry: That's a shocker. Many of us don't even know what our body is telling us. Maybe it's full from overindulging at the lunch buffet. Key is to take a few minutes and listen to your body. No guilt or shame required.

Stop for a few minutes: If you find yourself unconsciously going to the fridge to numb feelings of loneliness, sadness, anger or frustration, stop. Put a reminder on your fridge to stop and take a few breaths before you indulge. Tap into your feelings, and maybe instead of food you really need a hug or social connection such as calling a friend or loved one.

New Food Habits

Once you bring awareness to your actions around food, you can make small steps each day to form new habits. A good rule of thumb is to eat a mostly plant-based diet. Half your plate should be comprised of fruits and veggies. One quarter should be whole grains — or if you have gluten intolerance — gluten-free grains. The remaining quarter should be mostly plant-based protein. Also include water and fats and oils.[7]

It's good to remember that one person's poison is another person's medicine. While some people feel fine on a mostly plant-based diet, other people (especially if you are a blood type O) feel better with a little more animal protein. Make sure your meat is organic and grass fed and your fish is wild-caught and sustainable. Sticking to the mostly plant-based approach will increase your fertility. Key is to be kind to yourself and take small steps each day.

What Is the Best Place to Start?

This step is critical. Record what is going into your mouth every day. When you track it, you bring awareness to your actions around food. A lot of the time we eat unconsciously. It is not about calorie counting, but figuring out what your body is telling you and identifying cravings.

It always seems impossible until it's done.
—Nelson Mandela

You didn't gain or lose the weight overnight. It takes time to incorporate new, healthy eating habits. Refer to the crowding-out principle[8]. Eat a salad before lunch and dinner. Drink a glass of water if you feel hungry. Remember to practice self-care and refer back to the stress-reducing techniques.

What You Need To Know

- Losing 5% to 10% of your weight is enough to improve ovulation.
- Body mass index (BMI) above 30, which is considered obese, and BMI between 25 and 29.9, which is considered overweight, increases the risk of ovulatory infertility.
- Obese and overweight men have lower sperm counts or no sperm counts.
- Women with low BMI (below 19) have increased risk of miscarriage, and men with a low BMI have lower sperm counts.
- Eat mindfully. Slow down. Chew your food. Minimize your distractions.
- Get a food diary, and track what goes into your mouth.

From Your Coach
What are your thoughts about your weight?
You have been underweight/overweight your whole life? How will you change? It's in the genes; your whole family is underweight/overweight. You know that weight is affected by fertility, but it is so difficult when those cravings hit. Time to get curious with your thoughts. Remember, no judgment; grab your journal and start to write.

What may be holding you back from losing or gaining weight?
Sometimes we have limiting beliefs that we will never lose/gain weight. Maybe you have been overweight or underweight your whole life. Start to question those beliefs. You may even feel overwhelmed by all the decisions that need to be made. Remember, these thoughts and emotions are completely normal.

What is one step you can take to lose or gain weight?
Nourish your body with healthy whole grains, fruits and vegetables. Start each meal with a salad. Drink a glass of water when a craving hits. Commit to one step today.

Who will support you?
Partner, friend or coach.

Visualize a healthy weight for your body.
You feel empowered and good in your body. You look and feel vibrant and energized.

What Is Next?
Could vitamins impact your fertility?

Handy Resources
Website to help you calculate your BMI
http://www.nhlbi.nih.gov/health/educational/lose_wt/BMI/bmicalc.htm
Online apps and food diaries
http://www.redbookmag.com/health-wellness/advice/my-food-diary#slide-9

References
1. *http://www.jstor.org/discover/10.2307/3702368?uid=3739448&uid=2&uid=3737720&uid=4&sid=21104379282347*
2. *http://humupd.oxfordjournals.org/content/10/3/267.short*
3. *http://www.biomedcentral.com/content/pdf/1477-7827-1-109.pdf*
4. *http://www.hsph.harvard.edu/news/hsph-in-the-news/excess-weight-sperm-fertility/*
5. *http://humrep.oxfordjournals.org/content/23/4/878.short*
6. *http://www.sciencedirect.com/science/article/pii/S0015028204022241*
7. Institute for Integrative Nutrition – Food Plate, 2012
8. Institute for Integrative Nutrition, Crowding Out, 2012

Seventeen

VITAMINS AND
MINERALS

Now that you know how weight impacts fertility, let's switch gears and talk about supplements. The Harvard Nurses' Health Study found that regular use of multivitamins reduced the risk of ovulatory infertility.[6] The key ingredients that made the biggest contribution were folic acid and iron.

Folic Acid

Folic acid supplements help to reduce early miscarriages and pre-eclampsia (high blood pressure during pregnancy).

Food Sources for folic acid include lentils, pinto beans, chick-peas, asparagus, spinach, black beans, navy beans, kidney beans and collard greens.

Iron

The source of iron mattered. Women who got most of their iron from meat were not protected against ovulatory infertility. Those who got their iron from plant sources such as fruits, vegetables and beans increased their chances of getting pregnant.

Food sources of iron are spinach, tomatoes and lima beans.

Multivitamins

A multivitamin with extra folic acid dramatically reduces a woman's chances of having a baby with neural tube defects such as spina bifida.[7]

For men a multivitamin is good idea too. Not only does it show support for your partner by taking the daily supplement with her, but nutritional therapies have been proven to improve male fertility.[8]

Coenzyme Q10

Coenzyme Q10 is an antioxidant that is produced naturally by the body and is available as a supplement. It functions as an antioxidant, decreasing damage on the reproductive system. One study found that coenzyme Q10 increased sperm motility.[11] Another study found an increase in sperm count.[12] A study in the *Journal of Fertility and Sterility* found that older women taking 600 milligrams of coenzyme Q10 experienced improvement in both egg quality and fertilization rates.[13]

Food sources include spinach, kale, broccoli, nuts, meat and seafood.

Vitamin C

For men the most important vitamins for male fertility is vitamin C, along with the mineral zinc. Vitamin C helps reduce agglutination (or sperm sticking together), which is when antibodies are formed against the sperm.[1] Vitamin C also increases sperm count. In one study, when healthy men decreased their vitamin C from 250 milligrams to 5 milligrams a day, there was 91% increase in the number of sperm with damaged DNA.

Food sources of vitamin C are red and green peppers, broccoli, cabbage and Brussels sprouts.

Zinc

Men who are low in zinc may have infertility, but adding zinc can improve the sperm count. Zinc is one of the most important trace minerals for male infertility. It has been shown to boost sperm levels. Zinc is an important nutrient the body uses to produce testosterone. In one study zinc and folic acid taken together demonstrated a 74% increase in total normal sperm count.[3]

Sesame seeds, pumpkin seeds, lentils, cashews, walnuts, almonds, chickpeas, tempeh and tofu are good sources of zinc.

The best bet is to get all your nutrients from whole foods. When you eat whole foods, vitamins aren't really needed. But watch out. The billion-dollar vitamin industry wants you to take lots of supplements. If you decide to add supplements to boost your fertility, your local health food store has the best options. Brands such as New Roots, Natural Factor and Sisu are good brands. Alternatively, you can try Juice Plus from a representative. These are whole food supplements.

Probiotics

A probiotic is especially necessary for anyone battling candida. The probiotic will restore the health of your gut. The probiotic supplies friendly bacteria such as acidophilus and bifidus, which fight candida and its overgrowth. The friendly bacteria can also be found in yogurt, however many of the mass-produced yogurts do not have enough of the bacteria that you need.

You can use a powder or a supplement. You can dissolve the powder in a green juice, smoothie or water (wait a few minutes before you drink the water and it will completely dissolve). Alternatively, you can make your own sauerkraut or buy a brand such as Bubbies (in refrigerated section of your health food store). You should eat about 1 to 2 tablespoons per day to keep the bacteria in your gut healthy.

Vitamin D

As you may be aware, anyone living north of the equator may be deficient in vitamin D. This can lead to porous bones, fractures and osteoporosis. There is growing evidence that vitamin D protects against many forms of cancer. Vitamin D deficiency has also been linked to an increased risk of autism in children.[4] Vitamin D is important in repairing DNA damage and protecting against oxidative stress, so men too should ensure their levels are normal.

Also, if you go out in the sun between noon and 2 p.m. for about 10 minutes (with no sunscreen and no sunglasses) you will achieve the same affect.

Food Sources of vitamin D include dairy, soy, eggs, fatty fish and cod liver oil. During the 10-day challenge, these sources may not be an option, given that some people are intolerant to soy.

Omega-3s

Long-chain omega-3 fatty acids are eicosapentaenoic acid (EPA) and docosahexaenoic acid (DHA).[9] Both DHA and EPA have anti-inflammatory effects. DHA plays and important role in brain function and joint health. EPA regulates inflammation, the immune system, blood clotting and circulation. Omega-3 fatty acids are crucial to consume while trying to conceive. It is important for your baby's neural development and for preventing postpartum depression.[5]

Excellent Plant Sources for Omega-3s

- chia seed
- hemp seed or oil
- flax seed (ground) or oil (This can be a laxative to the body, so take with care if you experience any diarrhea or digestive upset.)
- microalgae oil
- afa algae (*Aphanizomenon flos-aquae*)
- marine phytoplankton
- walnuts

It's best to get all of your nutrients from food. However, studies have shown that fertility improves with the use of supplements.

What You Need to Know

- Regular use of a multivitamin reduces ovulatory infertility and boosts male fertility.
- Vitamin C and zinc are especially important for men.
- Daily probiotic is recommended to restore gut health, especially good for those with candida.
- Omega-3s are important for baby's neural development and preventing postpartum depression.

From Your Coach
What are your thoughts on vitamins?

You already eat a healthy diet, so why would you need them? You don't have time to take vitamins. You don't like the potential side effects. You know that they can impact your fertility. Time to get curious with your thoughts. Remember, no judgment; grab your journal and start to write.

What may be holding you back from taking vitamins?

They are too expensive. You don't know when in the day you will take them. You may even feel overwhelmed by all the decisions that need to be made. Remember, these thoughts and emotions are completely normal.

What is one step you can take to add vitamins to your daily routine?

How about adding it to an existing routine? For example, after you brush you teeth, take your vitamins. Commit to one step today.

Who will support you?

Partner, friend or coach.

Visualize your body being fueled with the beneficial effects of vitamins.
Envision feeling vibrant, healthy and energetic.

What Is Next?
How do herbs and nutritional supplements support your fertility?

Handy Resources
Make sure your multivitamin includes the following, according to Victoria Maizes, MD.

http://victoriamaizesmd.com/preparing-for-pregnancy/supplements/

Information on Juice Plus, a whole food supplement

http://www.juiceplus.com/content/JuicePlus/en/what-is-juice-plus.html.html#.Uh4l26DQnzI

Here is my favourite probiotic, Genestra HMF Super Powder.

http://www.amazon.com/Genestra-HMF-Super-Powder-4-2/dp/B003IGF20Q/ref=sr_1_1?ie=UTF8&qid=1382128306&sr=8-1&keywords=hmf+powder

Benefits of vitamin D, according to Dr. Andrew Weil

http://www.drweil.com/drw/u/ART02812/vitamin-d

References
1. *http://onlinelibrary.wiley.com/doi/10.1111/j.1749-6632.1987.tb23770.x/abstract;jsessionid=A3AEDABEBE2D7E584E01AB07A79E9324.f04t03?deniedAccessCustomisedMessage=&userIsAuthenticated=false*
2. *http://www.pnas.org/content/88/24/11003.short*
3. *http://www.sciencedirect.com/science/article/pii/S0015028201032290*
4. *http://www.sciencedirect.com/science/article/pii/S0306987709005301*
5. *http://healthyomega3.com/?s=postpartum+depression*

6. *http://www.sciencedirect.com/science/article/pii/ S001502820700828X*
7. *http://jama.jamanetwork.com/article.aspx?articleid=379576*
8. *http://europepmc.org/abstract/MED/10696117*
9. *http://www.webmd.com/diet/features/ what-to-know-about-omega-3s-and-fish*
10. *http://www.fertstert.org/article/S0015-0282(08)00487-1/abstract*
11. *http://www.fertstert.org/article/S0015-0282(08)00487-1/abstract*
12. *http://onlinelibrary.wiley.com/doi/10.1002/j.1939-4640.1994. tb00504.x/abstract*
13) *http://www.fertstert.org/article/S0015-0282(09)02484-4/ abstract*

Eighteen

HERBS AND NUTRITIONAL SUPPLEMENTS

We discovered how important vitamins can be for your fertility. What about herbs and nutritional supplements? Herbs can be an important part of boosting and supercharging fertility. It is important to consult with your health practitioner before starting any herbal remedy. As well, many herbs have not been sufficiently studied to know their full benefits or interactions.

Herbs
These herbs are recommended to boost fertility.

Ashwagandha

- helps with stress
- immune support
- helps with fatigue
- hormone balancer

Note: Do not take if your are pregnant or breastfeeding. It may lower blood sugar levels. It may decrease blood pressure. If you have multiple sclerosis, lupus, rheumatoid arthritis or other autoimmune conditions, it is best to avoid, as may cause the immune system to become more active.[10]

Vitex agnus-castus (chasteberry)

- regulates menstrual cycle
- helps with PMS symptoms
- supports normal hormonal balance
- encourages ovulation
- normalizes progesterone levels
- good for endometriosis

Note: Avoid if pregnant or breastfeeding or taking birth control pill. Side effects include nausea, mild gastrointestinal complaints, fatigue, menstrual disorders, dry mouth and acne.

Maca

- female hormone balance
- menstrual regulation
- enhances sexual desire in men and women
- increases fertility
- promotes normal sperm health

Note: Talk to your healthcare provider if you have any hormone-sensitive conditions such as breast cancer, uterine cancer, ovarian cancer, endometriosis or uterine fibroids. Extracts from maca might act like estrogen. If you have any condition that might be made worse by exposure to estrogen, do not use these extracts.[2] Avoid if pregnant or breast feeding. Take in powder form and add to your morning smoothie or take as capsule.

Tribulus Terrestris (Bulgarian grown)

- enhances sex drive and sexual performance in men
- increases sperm production
- helps with erectile dysfunction and antisperm antibodies
- encourages ovulation[13]
- good for PCOS[13]

Note: Avoid if pregnant or breastfeeding. May make prostate problems worse. May affect blood sugar levels.[14]

Panax Ginseng

- erectile dysfunction
- increases sperm count and motility

Note: May increase or decrease blood pressure. May lower blood sugar levels.

Dong Quai

- supports a normal menstrual cycle
- aids with PMS and occasional menstrual irregularities
- infertility
- premature ejaculation

Note: May cause sun sensitivity. Pregnant women and breastfeeding women should not take this supplement.

Licorice Root

- in the herbal form shakuyaku-kanzo-to, increases fertility in women with PCOS

Note: Large amounts can lead to water retention and thus increase blood pressure. Avoid if you have high blood pressure. Avoid during pregnancy.[5]

Maitake

- may induce ovulation in patients with PCOS [9]

Note: No known side effects.

Nutritional Supplements

Evening Primrose Oil

- balances hormones
- increases cervical mucus (Cervical mucus is necessary for all the sperm to move freely through the cervix.)
- reduces PMS symptoms

Note: Side effects include digestive upset. People with epilepsy should take with guidance of a physician. Best taken in conjunction with omega-3 fatty acids such as fish and flaxseed.[5]

Natural Progesterone Cream

- helps with symptoms of PMS
- good for PCOS and endometriosis (estrogen-dominant conditions)
- balances estrogen, regulates menses and relieves pain
- infertility
- ovarian cysts

Note: Natural progesterone cream has a good safety record. Women with a history of cancer should consult with a physician before using it. Women using birth control or synthetic progestin should avoid it.

L-arginine

- amino acid shown to increase sperm quality and count
- infertility
- helps with erectile dysfunction

Note: Arginine may interact with certain medications that lower blood pressure. It may also interact with certain heart medications and drugs such as Viagra that treat erectile dysfunction. Pregnant women and women who are nursing should not use.[6]

Royal Jelly

- energy booster
- immune booster

- PMS symptoms
- balances hormones

Note: Royal jelly is a substance that worker bees secrete to feed the queen bee. It contains B vitamins and other nutrients. Do not use if pregnant or breastfeeding. If there is a history of asthma or allergies, do not use, as it may cause serious reactions, even death. Do not use if you are allergic to bee pollen or honey. [11]

Bee Pollen

- boosts immunity
- reduces allergies (hay fever)
- fertility booster for both men and women

Note: It is one of the most nutrient-dense foods you can eat. It contains proteins, minerals and vitamins. If you are allergic to bee stings, you should avoid bee pollen. To make sure you are not allergic to bee pollen products, try a tiny amount first on the skin or tip of the tongue before beginning a regular dosage.[5] Not recommended for pregnant or breastfeeding women. Possible side effects include shortness of breath, hives, swelling and anaphylaxis (a life-threatening allergic reaction).[12]

Herbs and natural supplements can be a vital part of your super-charging fertility plan. Exercise caution, and always consult your health practitioner before beginning any herbs or nutritional supplements.

What You Need to Know

- There are many herbs and nutritional supplements that help with ovulation, PCOS, hormonal balance, sperm counts and erectile dysfunction.

- Before using a herb or nutritional supplement, consult your healthcare practitioner.

From Your Coach
What are your thoughts on herbs and nutritional supplements?
You were not aware they could help with your fertility. This may be something to explore. What about the side effects? Remember, no judgment; grab your journal and start to write.

What is holding you back from taking the herbs and nutritional supplements?
You don't need extra help. You are fine with whole foods. You don't believe the science supports their use. There are too many options. You may feel overwhelmed by all the decisions that need to be made. Remember, these thoughts and emotions are completely normal.

What is one step you will take today to add herbs and nutritional supplements to your diet?
Speak with your naturopath or certified herbalist. Commit to one the step today.

Who will support you?
Partner, friend or coach.

Visualize being healed by the natural properties of herbs and nutritional supplements.
Envision having enhanced fertility.

What Is Next?
Could something possibly get in your way of success?

Handy Resources
Botanical medicine for women's health

*http://www.amazon.ca/Botanical-Medicine-Womens-Health-1e/
dp/0443072779*

References

1. *http://www.askdrjj.com/Books_image/dugoua-safety-efficacy-
chastetree.pdf*
2. *http://www.webmd.com/vitamins-supplements/ingredientmono-
555-maca.aspx?activeingredientid=555&activeingredientname=maca*
3. *http://humrep.oxfordjournals.org/content/17/9/2287.short*
4. *http://www.webmd.com/vitamins-supplements/ingredientmono-
760-progesterone.aspx?activeingredientid=760&activeingredientnam
e=progesterone*
5. Prescription for Natural Cures
6. *http://www.webmd.com/heart/
arginine-heart-benefits-and-side-effects*
7. *http://www.webmd.com/vitamins-supplements/ingredientmono-
936-dong+quai.aspx?activeIngredientId=936&activeIngredientName
=dong+quai&source=1*
8. *http://www.webmd.com/vitamins-supplements/ingredientmono-
881-licorice.aspx?activeIngredientId=881&activeIngredientName=lic
orice&source=1*
9. *http://online.liebertpub.com/doi/abs/10.1089/acm.2009.0696*
10. http://www.webmd.com/vitamins-supplements/ingredientmo-
no-953-ashwagandha.aspx?activeingredientid=953&activeingredie
ntname=ashwagandha
11. *http://www.webmd.com/vitamins-supplements/ingredientmono-
503-royal+jelly.aspx?activeIngredientId=503&activeIngredientName
=royal+jelly&source=1*
12. *http://www.webmd.com/balance/
bee-pollen-benefits-and-side-effects*

13. *http://promedics.explorewebdev.com/site/downloads/Phytoptherapy%20for%20PCOS.pdf*

14. *http://www.webmd.com/vitamins-supplements/ingredientmono-39-tribulus.aspx?activeingredientid=39&activeingredientname=tribulus*

Nineteen

SELF-SABOTAGE

B efore we begin, a little word about self-sabotage. Here are some thoughts that may come up during the 10-day challenge.

- Whose idea was this natural fertility program anyway?
- Maybe this was a mistake.
- I can't keep this up. How can I follow through with these recommendations?
- Who am I to invest time and money in myself?
- What about everyone else? I need to keep them happy?

If any of these statements resonate with you, great, because where you are right now is exactly where you are supposed to be.

I share with my clients that self-sabotage rears its ugly little head a few times along the journey to wellness and any kind of change. The first time it rears its head is before you decide to commit. You make a list of excuses of why you don't need a program to boost your fertility. You already know what to do, and you don't need any help, thank you very much!

Thing is, if you could do it alone, you already would have done it.

The next time is about two weeks into the program. The honeymoon phase is over, and it starts to get a little more difficult.

Everything takes so much time to figure out. You want to go back to your old routine. You want to figure out how you can stop the program and give up. You are sick of being so "good." Just so you know, that's self-sabotage taking you off track again.

Realize that where you are on the journey is completely normal. When thoughts come up that want to take you off track, bring awareness to the thought. Once you bring it to the surface and take yourself off automatic pilot, you can create real, lasting change. Refer back to your intention that you set at the beginning of the book. Better yet, place your intention in a place that you can see every day. No one said it would be easy, but I'm telling you it will be worth it.

10 Steps on Your Journey to Fertility and Health
Step 1: review: Look over again the meal plan and pantry essential list.

Step 2: prepare your shopping list and purchase the ingredients.
You may want to have the same breakfast or lunch every day to keep it simple. Try the Fabulously Fertile Smoothie for breakfast and a salad for lunch. Mix it up with a different dinner. You can also have leftovers for lunch the next day.

Step 3: keep a food diary. This step is critical. Record what is going into your mouth every day. When you track it, you bring awareness to your actions around food. A lot of the time we eat unconsciously. This step is a key to your success. It is not about calorie counting, but figuring out what your body is telling you and identifying cravings.

Step 4: get your sleep and rest. Go to bed and get up and the same time every day. Take some time every day to get quiet. It can be as simple as taking one minute to listen to your breath or spending a few minutes meditating. Or you could practice the visualization

FABULOUSLY FERTILE

exercises. Take all technology out of your bedroom, and take one day per week to be completely technology free.

Step 5: get your running shoes and exercise clothes ready. You will aim for 30 minutes of exercise per day. If you don't regularly exercise, start with 5 to 10 minutes of walking each day, and build as you go. Better to start small than to overdo it.

Step 6: plan to stay hydrated. Get a water bottle, glass or stainless steel. Use a Brita or other water filter. Aim for at least eight glasses of filtered water per day.

Step 7: refer to your intention often. This is your "why" for super-charging your fertility. You may have been through years of infertility or miscarriage, or you simply want to get your body ready to have a baby. Take small steps every day. If you have doubt, take the next small step.

> *You were given this life because you were strong enough to live it.*
> —Author Unknown

Step 8: slow down. When you feel overwhelmed, take a deep breath and know that, as Bruno Mars says, "You are amazing just the way you are."

Step 9: consult your doctors. Before you begin the 10-day challenge, you may want to consult with your physician or other health-care practitioners.

Step 10: call on me. Join my Facebook page for daily tips and motivation:

149

https://www.facebook.com/sesacoaching. Or follow me on twitter: https://twitter.com/SesaCoaching. Or email me if you need support or would like to enroll in one of my customized coaching programs at *sarah.clark@sesacoaching.ca.*

Part 2

THE FABULOUSLY
FERTILE 10-DAY
CHALLENGE

INTRODUCING FOOD AFTER THE 10-DAY CHALLENGE

When the 10-day challenge is complete, you can begin to rechallenge some of the foods or you can keep them out of your diet for three months. The choice is up to you. Remember, it takes 90 days for the egg to renew itself, and the life cycle of sperm is 70 to 80 days. This is your chance to reset your diet, while you have the momentum of the 10-day challenge. The longer you stay with the recommendations, the better your body will have to boost its fertility naturally. You can always add two or three meat or fish options to your diet each week, or you may feel better with a plant-based diet. The choice is up to you.

Rechallenging Plan
Here is a sample plan if you opt to rechallenge the foods and determine if you have an intolerance.

Rechallenging Gluten

- Start with one food and try for three days.
- Wait for five days to try new food.
- Select one food such as whole wheat pasta.
  - Day 1: eat for lunch and dinner.
  - Day 2: eat for lunch and dinner.
  - Day 3: eat for lunch and dinner.

- Record how you feel both mentally and physically with the food. A food diary is essential.
- Watch out for delayed reactions, sometimes three or four days later or longer.
- Give your body time to adjust if there were any reactions.
- Wait until the following week to rechallenge dairy.

Rechallenging Dairy

- Select one food such as whole milk or cheese (pick only one).
  - Day 8: eat or drink for breakfast and lunch.
  - Day 9: eat or drink for breakfast and lunch.
  - Day 10: eat or drink for breakfast and lunch.
- Record how you feel both mentally and physically with the food. A food diary is essential.
- Watch out for delayed reactions, sometimes three or four days later or longer.

If you determine that you have a food intolerance, you may be relieved that you finally know how food is affecting your body, or you may be fearful that you will have nothing left to eat. In the beginning it can be difficult as you adjust to a new way of thinking about food. Know that you are not alone. I have customized meal plans with delicious mouth-watering recipes. As you begin to fuel your body with real food, watch as your health begins to soar. When you take small steps every day, this amounts to big change.

A journey of a thousand miles begins with a single step.

—Lao-tzu

EQUIPMENT AND SUPPLIES NEEDED

Equipment

Juicer

This is not essential, as you can use a blender to blend your green vegetables and drink the pulp. If you do not wish to consume the pulp, you can strain the vegetables through a fine-mesh sieve and then strain again through cheesecloth. The choice is up to you.

There are centrifugal juicers, cold-pressed juicers and masticating juicers. Centrifugal juicers are great for anyone new to juicing. They work quickly but don't juice sprouts, wheatgrass or nuts well. The cold-pressed and masticating juicers are more money but great for someone who plans to juice frequently. They yield less pulp. Downside is they have more parts to clean. Try Breville or Jack LaLanne models for both types of juicers.

Blender/Mixer

A high-speed blender is best such as Vitamix blender, Ninja or Blendtec. An upright countertop blender will work, but it may take longer to mix and combine the foods.

An immersion blender is a handheld kitchen appliance that purées food. This is good if you don't love certain veggies. You can blend them up so you don't see them. It is also great for puréeing soups.

A handheld mixer is great for baking. It is essential for mixing, blending, whipping and beating.

Pantry Essentials
These are some items that are good to keep in stock. Best to shop at Goodness Me, Whole Foods, Bulk Barn (has great gluten-free section) and health food section of your favourite grocery store.

Flour and Baking Items

- all-purpose gluten-free flour
- gluten-free rolled oats
- guar gum or xanthan gum
- psyllium husk

Bread
Best bread is from a gluten-free bakery. You must either freeze or keep at room temperature. Refrigeration causes bread to crumble. If you have candida, look for yeast-free options.

Grocery Store Options
These are usually in the freezer section:

- Vege-Hut: yeast/vegan/gluten-free
- Udi's Gluten-Free bread

Protein
Beans
- black beans: canned BPA free (organic) or dried
- lentils: canned BPA free (organic) or dried
- chickpeas: canned BPA free (organic) or dried
- tempeh: fermented soy

Bars

Only consume if you are in a pinch.

- GoMacro: *www.gomacro.com*
- Kind: *www.kindsnacks.com*

Cereal

Nature's Path: sugar-free puffed grain cereals

Dairy Alternatives

Pick your favourite milk alternative.

- Earth Balance: butter alternative
- coconut milk: unsweetened
- hemp milk: unsweetened
- rice milk: unsweetened
- almond milk: unsweetened

Grains

- quinoa
- short grain brown rice
- long grain brown rice
- brown jasmine rice

Oil

- olive oil
- coconut oil

- grapeseed oil
- vegetable oil
- sesame oil
- walnut oil

Pasta/Noodles

- brown rice pasta
- quinoa pasta
- amaranth pasta

Other

- black pepper
- Braggs unpasteurized apple cider vinegar
- brown rice vinegar
- Bubbies sauerkraut: natural probiotic in the refrigerated section
- egg replacer: egg substitute
- gluten-free vanilla
- tamari sauce: gluten-free soy sauce
- sea salt or pink Himalayan salt
- unsweetened shredded coconut
- Veganaise: vegan mayonnaise
- vegetable stock: organic

Herbs/Spices

- basil
- bay leaves
- cinnamon

- chives
- chili powder
- chili flakes
- cilantro
- cumin
- curry
- dill
- ginger: fresh or ground
- nutmeg
- parsley
- tumeric

Nuts and Nut Butter

- almonds
- almond butter
- cashews
- cashew butter
- macadamia butter
- tahini
- walnuts

Sea Vegetables

- dulse
- wakame

Seeds

- pumpkin seeds

- flax seeds: ground
- sunflower seeds
- sesame: white/black

Sweeteners

- unsweetened apple sauce
- brown rice syrup
- maple syrup: organic
- honey
- stevia: liquid or powdered (for baking)

Tea

- Celestial Seasonings
- Stash Tea Company

FABULOUSLY FERTILE 10-DAY CHALLENGE MEAL PLAN

Day 1

Day 2

Day 3

Day 4

.

RECIPES

BREAKFAST

Fabulously Fertile Smoothie

This smoothie is loaded with fertility superfoods. It can be your go-to morning smoothie. It is great for boosting egg health and helps with hormonal balance. The chia seeds are a complete source of protein and fibre. If you are going through IVF treatments, consult with your doctor whether it is appropriate to use maca, royal jelly or bee pollen.

Prep time: 5 minutes
Yield: 2 servings

1 cup frozen or fresh organic berries (blueberries, raspberries, cherries, blackberries)
1 cup spinach or kale, stems removed, washed
2 cups unsweetened almond, hemp milk or coconut milk
2 tablespoons chia seeds soaked in ½ cup of unsweetened nondairy milk for 10 minutes for gel to form (See note below.)
2 tablespoons maca powder
2 teaspoons cinnamon
2 teaspoons royal jelly (If allergic to bees, do not use.)
1 tablespoons bee pollen (If allergic to bees, do not use.)

- Mix ingredients in a high-speed blender. If mixture is too thick, add more nondairy milk.
- Serve immediately.

Notes

- If you suffer from thyroid issues, omit the spinach and kale. If you have allergies or asthma, do not use royal jelly or bee pollen.
- For the chia seeds, if you don't have time for soaking, throw the chia seeds in the smoothie without soaking. They will take a few minutes to expand while in the smoothie.

Tropical Delight Smoothie

This smoothie is full of fertility-boosting ingredients such as maca and royal jelly. Pineapple contains bromelain, which has been shown to help with the pain associated with endometriosis. Coconut milk is especially good for candida, as it has antimicrobial properties to fight the yeast.

Prep time: 5 minutes
Yield: 2 servings

1/4 cup pineapple, chopped
½ cup mango, chopped
½ cup strawberries, chopped
1 banana
2 cups coconut milk
2 tablespoons unsweetened coconut
2 tablespoons maca
2 teaspoons royal jelly

- Combine ingredients in a high-speed blender, and blend.
- Serve immediately.

Note

- If you have candida, substitute banana, mango and pineapple for raspberries, blueberries and ¼ cup Thai coconut milk (full-fat version from can) to make it creamy.

Tip

- Save canned coconut milk in the refrigerator to add to your smoothie the next day.

Chocoholic Delight Smoothie

This smoothie is for chocoholics, but it doesn't have sugar and dairy like regular milk chocolate. It satisfies chocolate cravings but is loaded with magnesium. Keep your consumption to a minimum, as cocao does contain caffeine. See note at bottom regarding caffeine.

Prep time: 5 minutes
Yield: 2 servings

1 avocado, peeled and sliced
1 banana, peeled and chopped
2 tablespoons cocao powder
2 ½ cups unsweetened almond milk or rice milk
2 tablespoons maple syrup

- Combine ingredients in high-speed blender.
- Serve immediately.

Notes

- If you have candida, omit the banana, and add 1 ½ cups of unsweetened almond milk or rice milk – add more liquid to achieve desired thickness
- If you have candida and/or PCOS, omit maple syrup and add 2–3 drops of stevia to achieve desired sweetness.
- Cocoa does have caffeine, and studies advise that any more than 200 milligrams or 2 cups of coffee is not advised if you are trying to conceive.
- Each tablespoon of cocoa powder has 12 milligrams of caffeine.

Berry Berry Smoothie

I love this smoothie when I am running out the door and don't have time for breakfast. It's filling and doesn't require much time to prepare. The probiotic helps to restore gut flora and prepare your body for conception.

Prep time: 5 minutes
Yield: 2 servings

2 cup berries (blueberries, raspberries, blackberries), fresh or frozen
1 cup baby spinach
2 cup unsweetened almond milk or coconut milk
¼ cup almond butter
½ teaspoon cinnamon
2 tablespoons hemp seeds
2 tablespoons unsweetened shredded coconut
2 scoops of probiotic (HMF powder) (See tip.)
2 or 3 pitted dates, soaked for 30 minutes (optional for added sweetness)

- Add ingredients to a high-speed blender. If mixture too thick, add more nondairy milk.
- Blend until ingredients are fully combined.
- Serve immediately.

Notes

- Omit the spinach if you have thyroid problems. Omit the almond butter if you have candida, and substitute 2 tablespoons chia seeds.

Tip

- You can purchase the HMF powder probiotic in the refrigerator section of your local health food store or vitamin store.

Apple Pie Smoothie
In Norse mythology (gods and goddesses loved by the Vikings) apples are associated with fertility and youth. This smoothie will give you the taste of your favourite apple pie without the added sugar.

Prep time: 5 minutes
Yield: 2 servings

2 apples (Granny Smith), cored and chopped (peel can be left on)
¼ cup gluten-free oatmeal flakes (dry)
2 cups unsweetened almond milk or nondairy milk
1 teaspoon cinnamon
½ teaspoons nutmeg
2 tablespoons maca
2 date (pitted)

- Combine ingredients in high-speed blender.
- Serve immediately.

Note

- if you have candida, omit the dates.

Giddy Up Green Juice

This is my go-to all time favourite juice. Better than a coffee for getting me going in the morning. If you like a more mellow flavour, use the romaine lettuce, or try kale if you want to rev it up. The green apple gives it a bit of sweetness. Omit if you don't mind the grassy flavour. This juice is great if you have candida. It balances hormones, cleanses the liver and promotes egg and sperm health.

Prep time: 5 minutes
Yield: 1–2 servings

1 head romaine lettuce, or 5–6 kale leaves (stems removed) if want stronger flavour
1 cucumber (peeled if not organic)
4 stalks of celery
1 green apple (Granny Smith), quartered
½ fresh lemon, squeezed (optional)
¼ teaspoon ginger, grated

- Wash all ingredients.
- Insert each ingredient one by one into the juicer.
- Squeeze the lemon into the juice.
- Add fresh ginger to taste.

Notes

- If you have thyroid problems, omit the kale.
- For optimal benefits, organic produce is always preferred.

Ch–Ch Chia Pudding
If you want to clear out your digestive tract and supercharge your morning, this pudding is for you. Chia is loaded with omega-3 fatty acids, antioxidants, fibre and protein. Toss it in the fridge overnight, and wake up to a perfect pudding. The walnuts and banana are fertility superfoods. The walnuts add additional omega -3 fatty acids to your morning, which combat inflammation, and the banana improves sperm quality.

Prep time: 5 minutes, chia seeds and milk to soak for 8–12 hours
Yield: 2 servings

6 tablespoons chia seeds
1 cup unsweetened almond milk or nondairy milk
1 banana, peeled and chopped
2 tablespoons walnuts, chopped
1 tablespoon maple syrup

- In medium bowl, combine chia seeds and almond milk.
- Place in refrigerator overnight, or wait 30–60 minutes, until seeds expand and form a gel.
- Add banana, walnuts and maple syrup.
- Serve and enjoy.

Notes

- If it is too gelatinous, you can pop the mixture in the blender for 30 seconds on high.
- If you have candida and/or PCOS, substitute maple syrup for 2–3 drops of stevia. Add more to achieve desired level of sweetness. Omit banana and substitute berries such as blueberries if you have candida.

Creamy Brown Rice Porridge

This creamy porridge can be eaten for breakfast or as a sweet treat. Brown rice is a slow carbohydrate. Slow carbohydrates minimize insulin resistance, regulate blood sugar, improve fertility and help prevent gestational diabetes.

Prep time: 15 minutes (if rice not cooked, 45 minutes)
Yield: 2 servings

3 cups brown rice, short or long grain, cooked
1 cup unsweetened almond milk or nondairy milk
1 tablespoon maple syrup
½ teaspoon cinnamon
2 tablespoons walnuts, chopped
2 tablespoons raisins or pitted dates, chopped
1 tablespoon unsweetened coconut

- In saucepan, add brown rice and almond milk or nondairy milk of your choice.
- Cover and heat for 7–10 minutes, or until warm.
- Remove from heat, and add cinnamon, walnuts, raisins or dates and coconut.
- Stir to combine.
- Serve immediately.

Notes

- if you have candida, eliminate raisins, dates and nuts, and substitute maple syrup for 2–3 drops of stevia. You can add ½ teaspoon nutmeg and ½ teaspoon of ginger for more flavour.

- If you have PCOS, substitute maple syrup for 2–3 drops of stevia.

Tip

- To prepare rice, take 1½ cups of uncooked brown rice (long or short grain) and combine with 3 cups of water. Cook according to package, typically 45 minutes. You can make extra too.

Nutty Raisin Cereal

This cereal will keep you full all morning long. It's loaded with omega-3 essential fatty acids such as walnuts that help to improve sperm quality. Cinnamon is great for inflammation and helps to reduce sugar cravings by controlling blood sugar levels. This is beneficial if you have PCOS.

Prep time: 5 minutes
Yield: 2 servings

1/3 cup walnuts, chopped
¼ cup unsweetened shredded coconut
¼ hemp hearts
1 tablespoon ground chia seeds
1 tablespoon ground cinnamon
¼ cup raisins, or dates or figs
¼ teaspoon sea salt
2 cups water

- In a high-powered blender, grind the walnuts, shredded coconut, hemp hearts, chia seeds and cinnamon, until smooth.
- Transfer mixture to a medium saucepan, and add water and raisins.
- Cook for 10 minutes.
- Serve immediately.

Note

- if you have candida, substitute walnuts for pumpkin seeds and eliminate raisins, dates and figs.

Gluten-Free French Toast With Blueberry Syrup
A gluten-free diet is great for clearing your (and your partner's) system to increase your pregnancy chances. According to studies, gluten can deplete nutrition, lower your immunity and cause inflammation. Bad news for pregnancy. The good news is that you can still enjoy your favourite breakfast meal! There are substitutes for everything, and here's one of them. Not only is this French toast wheat free, it is also cholesterol free and contains fibre, along with omega-3 fatty acids from flax seeds. For this recipe, it's best to make the syrup first so it will be ready for the hot French toast.

Prep time: 30 minutes
Yield: 2 servings

8 slices of gluten-free bread of your choice, cut diagonally
1 cup buckwheat flour, sifted
1 tablespoon flax seeds, ground
2 teaspoons ground cinnamon
½ teaspoon Himalayan sea salt (optional)
1 cup coconut milk
1 ripe banana, mashed
2 tablespoons maple syrup
1 teaspoon vanilla extract
¼ cup cold-pressed coconut oil for frying

Blueberry Syrup
1 cup blueberries, fresh or frozen
½ cup maple syrup

To Prepare Blueberry Syrup

- Using a blender, combine the maple syrup and ¾ cup of the blueberries.
- Stir in remaining whole blueberries, and set aside.

To Prepare French Toast

- In a bowl, mix together buckwheat flour, flax seeds cinnamon and sea salt.
- Stir in coconut milk, banana, maple syrup and vanilla extract.
- Heat 2 tablespoons of coconut oil in a skillet on medium heat.
- Dip one bread slice at a time into the batter, coating each side.
- Add 2–4 batter-coated slices of bread to the skillet, and cook on each side, until golden brown.
- Remove, and allow to cool on a plate or rack.
- Repeat with remaining slices.
- Serve with blueberry syrup and banana slices.

Notes

- If you have candida and/or PCOS, serve with fresh blueberries with 2–3 drops of stevia to taste.
- If you have candida, omit the banana from the batter and the topping. For the batter reduce coconut milk to ¾ cup.

SOUPS AND SALADS

Baby Carrot Soup

It's time to eat from the rainbow, starting with orange and yellow. These types of veggies contain an abundance of beta-carotene, which has been shown to maintain hormonal balance, prevent miscarriage and improve sperm motility.

Prep time: 25 minutes
Yield: 4 servings

2–3 large carrots, chopped small (See note if you have candida.)
1 onion, chopped small
1 teaspoon fresh ginger, minced
½ teaspoon cinnamon
½ teaspoon cumin
1½ teaspoons curry powder
1 ¾ cup vegetable broth
14-ounce can coconut milk
sea salt to taste

- In a large pot, simmer the carrots, onions, ginger, cinnamon, cumin and curry powder in vegetable broth for 20–25 minutes, until carrots are soft.
- Allow soup to cool slightly.
- Using either an immersion/handheld blender or upright blender, purée soup.
- Return to heat, and stir in coconut milk, until well combined.
- Season with sea salt to taste.

Note

- If you have candida, do not consume starchy vegetables such as carrots, as they are not tolerated during the first 3 weeks of the candida diet.

Triplet Noodle Tempeh Soup

Research has shown that a well-nourished woman is more likely to have a multiple birth. This hearty noodle soup will feed your body and your soul. It contains good-quality and easily digestible proteins, trace minerals and vegetable fat to boost your chances of conceiving. Tempeh is a fermented soy product. If you can get access to Indonesian-made tempeh, this recipe will be out of this world. Though it still tastes fantastic with regular tempeh;-). Rice noodles, kelp noodles and tempeh can all be purchased at Asian markets, health food stores and online. These noodles can also be substituted for other gluten-free noodles of your choice. Get that creative energy flowing!

Prep time: 30 minutes
Yield: 4 servings

4 cups of purified water
4 cups vegetable broth
2 cups coconut milk
2 scallions, thinly sliced
2 carrots, peeled and shredded fine
1 thumb-size piece of ginger, grated
1 cup unseasoned tempeh of your choice
2 tablespoons tamari
4 ounces/75 grams rice noodles
4 ounces/75 grams black rice noodles
4 ounces/75 grams kelp noodles (refrigerated section of grocery store)
3 tablespoons toasted sesame oil
sea salt to taste (optional)

- Cut tempeh into bite-sized pieces, and place in medium bowl. Add tamari, combine and set aside.

Marinate for 15 minutes.
- In a large pot, add water, vegetable broth and coconut milk, and bring to a boil.
- Add tempeh and remaining ingredients to the soup pot.
- Allow to boil for 10 minutes.
- If necessary, adjust flavours to your taste.
- Remove from heat and serve.

Tips

- It's always good to make extra soup to freeze.
- Substitute gluten-free noodles such as quinoa or amaranth

Warm and Cozy Butternut Soup
True story. One season, a kibbutz in southern Israel had an abundant squash crop on their organic farm. Nine months later, the community gave birth to a record number of twins. Squash is loaded with great fertility nutrients: beta-carotene, folate, vitamin C, potassium, omega-3 fatty acids and fibre. The brewer's yeast (aka nutritional yeast) — a naturally occurring nonactive dry yeast derived from beer — in this recipe is packed with vitamin B12, which is essential for healthy ovulation. It adds a great flavour to soups and main dishes. The homemade sesame seed milk is rich in calcium.

Prep time: 20 minutes
Cooking time: 30 minutes
Yield: 4 servings

Two 3–pound butternut squash, peeled, seeded and coarsely chopped (See note if you have candida.)
1 clove garlic, chopped
1 thumb-sized piece of ginger, grated
1 large yellow onion, chopped
1 cup cold-pressed extra virgin olive oil (includes 2 tablespoons for sautéing vegetables)
2 tablespoons fresh sage, chopped
½ teaspoon ground nutmeg
Himalayan sea salt to taste
8 cups vegetable stock

Sesame Seed Milk
¾ cup filtered water or enough water to cover the blender blades
¼ cup sesame seeds

- In a large pot, sauté the squash, garlic, ginger and

onions in 2 tablespoons of olive oil at a medium temperature for a few minutes, until slightly soft.

- Add sage, ground nutmeg and sea salt.
- Cook for another few minutes.
- Add vegetable stock. If it does not cover the squash, add some extra water.
- Bring the soup to a boil, and simmer for about 30 minutes.
- While the soup is boiling, prepare the sesame seed milk.
- Blend sesame seeds and water in a high-speed blender, until creamy. If milk is too thick, add more water. If too thin, add more sesame seeds. Pour in a bowl, and set aside.
- Fill blender ¾ full of soup. Holding the lid tightly, blend the soup, until smooth. (Be careful with glass blenders.) Pour soup back into the pot. Repeat until all soup is blended.
- Stir in 1 cup of sesame seed milk, nutritional yeast and remaining olive oil. Serve hot (or warm).

Notes

- If you have candida, do not consume starchy vegetables such as squash, as they are not tolerated during the first 3 weeks of the candida diet.

Tip

- If you have extra sesame seed milk, it is perfect to add to your smoothie.

Dipping Lentil Tomato Soup

This is a fast and easy weeknight dinner. My son likes to dip his bread in the lentil soup. Tomatoes are loaded with vitamin C, which builds connective tissue, keeps blood vessels healthy and boosts the immune system. Lentils are full of vitamin B9 and folate, which help reduce the risk of birth defects like spina bifida and cancer.

Prep time: 10 minutes
Cooking time: 20 minutes
Yield: 4 servings

1 tablespoons olive oil
1 onion, chopped
2 garlic cloves, minced
28-ounce can organic diced tomatoes
15-ounce can green lentils (See note if you have candida.)
2 cups vegetable stock
1 tablespoon cumin
1 teaspoon coriander seeds
1 bay leaf
sea salt and ground pepper to taste

- Heat oil in large stock pot over medium heat.
- Add onion, and sauté, until onion is translucent.
- Add garlic and sauté for 1–2 minutes.
- Stir in tomatoes, green lentils (or substitute chicken or turkey) and vegetable stock.
- Add cumin and coriander seeds, bay leaf, sea salt and pepper.
- Allow soup to boil, then simmer for 15–20 minutes.
- Serve with gluten-free bread for dipping!

Note

- If you have candida, avoid legumes for the first 3–4 weeks. Substitute lean protein such as 2 chicken or turkey breasts. Cut chicken or turkey into 1-inch pieces, and in a medium saucepan with 1 tablespoon of olive, sauté, until golden brown.

Creamy Cashew Tomato Soup
Raw soups are great for adding variety to your fertility diet. They are easily digestible, which is wonderful, since indigestion is a common complaint before, during and after the pregnancy process. I have found cashews to be one of the best bases for raw soups. Here's a pretty simple and tasty recipe. It is best to have a high-speed blender when preparing raw soup, but any blender will do.

Prep time: 15 minutes
Yield: 4 servings

2 cups cashews, soaked 8 hours, rinsed and drained
2 cups filtered water
2 Roma tomatoes, peeled
6 sundried tomatoes (not packed in oil), soaked (Reserve water.)
4 fresh basil leaves
1 garlic clove, pressed
½ teaspoon Himalayan sea salt (optional)

- Blend cashews and water in a high-speed blender.
- Add remaining ingredients, except for the water used for soaking sundried tomatoes.
- Blend until mixture is your desired soup consistency. Slowly add sundried tomato water if more liquid is needed.
- Serve immediately.

Notes

- if you have candida, omit cashews.
- Blending in the high-speed blender adds warmth to the soup, so it's best to eat it right away.
- Tastes great with flax seed crackers.

Taboulleh Baby

The calcium in the almonds helps strengthen your bones in preparation for conception and childbirth. Soaking the almonds helps the body to better absorb the nutrients. The chlorophyll in the green herbs is a great blood builder for your reproductive system. Olive oil and lemon juice are great for overall reproductive health.

Prep time: 30 minutes
Yield: 8 servings

1 bunch fresh flat leaf parsley, washed and large stems removed
6 scallions, white part removed
4 Roma tomatoes, peeled and seeded
2 tablespoons cold-pressed extra virgin olive oil
2 tablespoons fresh lemon juice
1 handful fresh mint leaves
¼ cup raw almonds, soaked for 8 hours, rinsed and coarsely ground

- Place all ingredients, except for the almonds, in the food processor and chop fine.
- Pour mixture into a bowl.
- Stir in almonds and serve.

Note

- If you have candida, omit the almonds.

Tutti–Fruitti Salad with Peanut Butter Sauce
This very flexible and filling fruit salad recipe can be adjusted according to taste. Add or delete whichever fruits you like. You can make the peanut butter sauce thicker, thinner, sweeter or nuttier. You can save extra sauce for an excellent protein shake.

Prep time: 10–15 minutes
Yield: 2 servings

4 bananas, sliced
4 apples (preferably pink lady), diced small (optional to remove peel)
½ cup dried mulberries (or dried figs, raisins, or dried cranberries)
2 tablespoons dried coconut (optional)

Peanut Butter Sauce (See note.)
½ cup peanut butter, organic
¼ cup maple syrup
filtered water

- Stir to combine peanut butter, maple syrup and water.
- Adjust amount of water, depending on desired thickness.

Notes

- If you have candida, omit banana and peanut butter sauce.
- If you have PCOS and/or candida, omit dried fruit and substitute 5–10 drops of stevia to taste.

Twins Cabbage Salad

This colorful raw food dish is energizing, cleansing and delicious. Cabbage contains a phytonutrient called Di-indole methane (DIM), which regulates estrogen, prevents fibroids and helps to prevent endometriosis. Cabbage loves your uterus. So why not get a double dose? You never know what might happen. (Wink! Wink!)

Prep time: 20 minutes
Yield: 6–8 servings

1 cup purple cabbage, shredded fine
1 cup green cabbage, shredded fine
1 large carrot, peeled and thinly sliced
1 large parsnip, peeled and thinly sliced
½ red bell pepper, seeded and thinly sliced into strips
½ green bell pepper, seeded and thinly sliced into strips
1 handful of cashews
¼ cup cold-pressed extra virgin olive oil
2 tablespoons unpasteurized apple cider vinegar (Braggs)
2 tablespoons maple syrup

- In a large bowl, thoroughly mix all ingredients.
- You can eat now, but it tastes best after marinating for an hour or so.

Notes

- if you have candida, omit cashews.
- If you have candida and/or PCOS, substitute maple syrup with 2–3 drops stevia to taste.

Chickpea and Tahini Salad
This is a fast lunch option that you can make ahead of time. The flavours will intensity overnight as you sleep. The sesame seeds in the tahini help to balance hormones in the body to block excess estrogen. Excess estrogen can cause irregular periods, anxiety, depression and digestive issues.

Prep time: 10 minutes
Yield: 2 servings

15-ounce can of chickpeas, rinsed and drained (Or substitute chicken or turkey.) (See note if you have candida.)
¼ cup fresh parsley, chopped
¼ cup red onion, finely chopped
½ cup cucumber, chopped
2 cloves garlic, minced
½ lemon, freshly squeezed
2 tablespoons olive oil
2 tablespoons tahini
Freshly ground pepper and sea salt

- In a medium bowl, combine chickpeas (or chicken or turkey if using), parsley, red onion and cucumber.
- In a small bowl, whisk together garlic, lemon, olive oil and tahini.
- Add the dressing mixture to the chickpea (or chicken or turkey if using) mixture, and combine.
- Season with salt and pepper to taste.

Notes

- If you have candida, avoid legumes for the first 3–4 weeks. Substitute lean protein such as 2 chicken or turkey breasts. Cut chicken or turkey into 1-inch pieces, and in a medium saucepan with 1 tablespoon of olive, sauté, until golden brown.

Spring Is in the Air Salad

This spring salad mix contains powerful herbs such as endive, dandelion and chervil, which strengthen the immune system in preparation for conception. This salad also contains essential nutrients such as blood-cleansing chlorophyll and nerve-nourishing vitamin B12. Avocados contain good fat that your body needs to carry the weight of a baby.

Prep time: 30 minutes, or 10 minutes (if using ready-made salad mix)
Yield: 8 servings

4 cups spring salad mix, gently torn (or if pressed for time, ready-made salad mix: endive, dandelion, chervil)
2 Roma tomatoes, sliced
1 carrot, shredded (See note if you have candida.)
1 cucumber, thinly sliced
2 tablespoons wakame seaweed, soaked and drained
2 tablespoons balsamic vinegar
1 avocado, peeled and diced
A dash of Himalayan sea salt to taste (optional)

- In a large bowl, mix all ingredients together and serve.

Notes

- Omit carrot, and substitute zucchini if you have candida.
- Wakame has a slightly "fishy" taste and smell, so you may like more or less on your salad. You can find it in the Asian section of your health food store.

Broccoli–ishous Salad

Time to get your greens. Green vegetables are essential for reproductive health. Broccoli is part of the cruciferous family. Cruciferous vegetables have high levels of phytochemicals that work to block estrogen production. This is beneficial for PCOS, endometriosis, uterine fibroids, ovarian cysts and low sperm count.

Prep time: 20 minutes
Yield: 4 servings

2 medium crowns or stalks of broccoli (about 4 cups)
2 scallions, chopped
2–3 tablespoons sunflower seeds
2–3 tablespoons raisins

For the Dressing
2 tablespoons Veganaise (mayonnaise substitute)
2 tablespoons lemon, freshly squeezed
1½ tablespoons olive oil or grapeseed oil
1 teaspoon red wine vinegar
1 teaspoon maple syrup
2–3 teaspoons Dijon mustard
freshly ground black pepper

- Cut off the stems from the broccoli, and cut into bite-sized pieces.
- Using a medium bowl, combine ingredients for the dressing, and whisk, until combined.
- Add broccoli, seeds, scallions and raisins.
- Toss to combine and serve.

Notes

- Do not consume if you have thyroid problems due to raw cruciferous vegetables, which inhibit the thyroid.
- If you have candida and/or PCOS, substitute maple syrup with 1-2 drops of stevia.
- If you have candida omit raisins.

Baby Kale Salad

This salad will send your taste buds soaring and get your baby house ready. The walnut oil is loaded with omega-3 fatty acids, which boost fertility. The dulse flakes have iodine, which is supportive for your thyroid. Aim for 2–3 servings of sea vegetables per week. Dulse contains 4 times more iron than spinach. The apple cider vinegar will help to fight candida by restoring gut flora.

Prep time: 20 minutes
Yield: 2 servings

For Chickpeas
15-ounce can chickpeas, rinsed and drained (Or substitute chicken or turkey.) (See note if you have candida.)
1 tablespoon olive oil
½ teaspoon sea salt
¼ teaspoon freshly ground black pepper

For the salad
4–6 cups baby kale, washed and patted dry
2 tablespoons dulse flakes
2 tablespoons pumpkin seeds
2 tablespoons walnut oil
1 tablespoon unpasteurized apple cider vinegar (Braggs)

- Preheat oven to 425° F. Line a baking sheet with aluminum foil. (Omit this step and the next step if you have candida. See note below.)
- Place the chickpeas on the prepared baking sheet, and toss with the olive oil, salt and pepper. Roast for 10–12 minutes, stirring once, until the chickpeas are slightly shrunken and crispy. Let cool.

- In a large bowl, combine the walnut oil and apple cider vinegar.
- Add the baby kale, and toss, until evenly coated.
- Add the roasted chickpeas (or chicken or turkey if using).
- Sprinkle with dulse flakes and pumpkin seeds.
- Serve immediately.

Note

- If you have candida, avoid legumes for the first 3–4 weeks. Substitute lean protein such as 2 chicken or turkey breasts. Cut chicken or turkey into 1-inch pieces, and in a medium saucepan with 1 tablespoon of olive, sauté, until golden brown.

Incredible Swiss Chard Callaloo

Pregnancy and giving birth can stress every part of your body, including your vision. (In fact, the stress and worry of *getting* pregnant can stress your vision.) Swiss chard contains the plant carotenoids lutein and zeaxanthin, which strengthen and protect your eyes. This recipe can be made with any of your favourite dark green leafy vegetables. I chose Swiss chard because it contains its own natural sodium for a great tasting salt-free dish. It is important to chop the vegetables right before cooking so they don't lose their juice as they sit.

Prep time and cook time: 40 minutes
Yield: 4 servings

1 bunch Swiss chard greens, thoroughly washed and finely shredded
1 yellow onion, finely chopped
1 medium tomato, diced small
2 garlic cloves, chopped
1 cup coconut milk
1 sprig of fresh thyme
1 Scotch bonnet pepper, finely chopped (optional) (See tip.)
1–2 tablespoons cold-pressed coconut oil

- In a skillet, sauté the garlic, onion and tomato with coconut oil for 5 minutes over medium heat.
- Add remaining ingredients and stir.
- Cook for 10 minutes, stirring occasionally.
- Turn down heat to low, and simmer for 15 minutes, or until greens are tender.

Tip

- Cut Scotch bonnet pepper using a knife and fork, being careful not to get the pepper on your hands, as it may sting. Never rub your eyes or touch your tongue or any other sensitive part of your body for up to 1 hour after handling the pepper.

Get Your Greens

Greens are an essential part of your everyday *Fabulously Fertile* meal plan. Switch up this recipe with kale, collard greens, Swiss chard and beet greens. The list is endless. Green vegetables supply the body with important vitamins and minerals such as beta-carotene and vitamin C.

Prep time: 10 minutes
Yield: 2 servings

1 tablespoon olive oil
2 garlic cloves, minced
4 cups baby spinach, washed
sea salt and black pepper to taste

- In a large frying pan on medium heat, add olive oil, and sauté the garlic for about 2 minutes.
- Add spinach, and cook, until it is wilted.

Note

- You can substitute the spinach for kale (wash, remove stems, roughly chop) and Swiss chard (wash, roughly chop).

Mineral-Rich Sauerkraut

Sauerkraut has excellent probiotic effects. This good bacteria is necessary for balanced colon health. Fermented foods are a necessary part of our diet. Most cultures have some form of fermented food in their daily diet to keep their health balanced. In North America, we tend to get little to no fermented foods in our diet and tend to suffer from constipation and vitamin and mineral deficiencies. These deficiencies tend to lead us on the path to other diseases and disorders such as infertility. Sauerkraut can be made salt free. Kelp and dulse add trace minerals for optimal health. The caraway seeds help alleviate indigestion.

Prep time: 20–25 minutes; fermentation: 3 days to 2 weeks
Yield: 4 servings

1 large head green cabbage
½ teaspoon sea salt (optional)
1 teaspoon granulated kelp
1 teaspoon granulated dulse
1 teaspoon caraway seeds
1 large Mason jar

- Discard outer leaves of cabbage. Cut the cabbage off the core.
- Using a food processor, cut cabbage into fine shreds.
- In a Mason jar, pack cabbage as tightly as you can, sprinkling salt and herbs between the layers. Eliminate as much air as possible.
- Keep the jar covered at all times with a cheesecloth.
- Store in a cool (55° F to 65° F) place for 3 days to 2 weeks.
- Each day check the sauerkraut, and press it down.

- As juice forms, use a small jelly jar filled with rocks or marbles to press down cabbage. It is important to keep cabbage submerged in its liquid.
- As white foam forms at the top, skim it off. This is part of the fermentation process.
- Taste the sauerkraut each day. When sauerkraut is ready (meaning that it tastes good to you, sour, kind of like a good pickle), store in a refrigerator to prevent spoilage.
- It lasts in the refrigerator for about 3 weeks.

Notes

- Sauerkraut will help restore gut flora, especially for those with candida. Aim for 2–3 tablespoons per day.
- Need some sauerkraut now, without the wait? My favourite is Bubbies. Sold in the refrigerator section of the health food store.

MAIN MEALS

Chickpea Mexican Burgers

Feel like having a fiesta? These burgers will get you in the mood to shake your maracas. Chickpeas have high protein and fibre content and are low in saturated fats. They have vitamin B6, which is essential for hormone regulation. Ginger is anti-inflammatory and helps to support the inflammatory symptoms associated with endometriosis. Cilantro is high in folic acid. What are you waiting for? Grab your partner and dance. Ole, Ole, Ole!

Prep time: 15–20 minutes
Cooking time: 12 minutes
Yield: 4 servings

15-ounce can chickpeas (See note if you have candida.)
1 cup short brown rice, cooked (See tip and note if you have candida.)
2 tablespoons tamari, sodium reduced
½ red onion, finely chopped
1 tablespoon ginger, ground
¼ cup cilantro, chopped
1 lime, freshly squeezed
freshly ground pepper and sea salt to taste
1 tablespoon olive oil

- In a medium bowl, combine all ingredients, mashing chickpeas with fork or potato masher to combine (Omit mashing step if have candida.)
- Form into 4 patties. Set aside.
- Preheat large skillet or frying pan, and add 1 tablespoon olive oil.

- Cook burgers for 6 minutes on each side, until lightly browned.
- Serve with gluten-free bun or Boston bibb lettuce wrap.

Notes

- If you have candida, avoid legumes for the first 3–4 weeks. Substitute lean protein such as 1 package (1 pound, or .45 kilogram) ground chicken or turkey. Omit brown rice.
- Combine ½ cup rice with 1 cup of water. This will give your approximately 1 cup of cooked rice.
- It's always best to cook more so you can use it in soups, salads and even throw it in your smoothie.

Powerful Parsley Pesto
Cauliflower is packed with vitamin C, fibre and folate. Cauliflower helps to balance out the hormones and boost sperm quality. The pasta helps to keep you full and prevent those nasty spikes in blood sugar like the white pasta does. Serve your pasta slightly el dente (or firm to the bite). If it is overcooked, it has a tendency to go mushy.

Prep time: 20 minutes
Cooking time: 7 minutes
Yield: 4 servings

2 cups flat leaf parsley sprigs
3 tablespoons capers, drained
1 lemon, zested and juiced
½ teaspoon crushed red pepper flakes to taste
3 garlic cloves, peeled
½ cup extra virgin olive oil
freshly ground pepper and sea salt to taste
16 ounces, or 454 grams, brown rice or quinoa pasta (penne or rigatoni)
2 cups cauliflower florets

- Place parsley, capers, lemon zest and juice, red pepper flakes, garlic and olive oil in a high-speed blender or food processor to combine.
- Bring large pot of water to boil, add pasta and cauliflower florets and cook for 7 minutes, or according to package.
- Serve immediately.

Sweet Lentils and Spinach

Compared to other dried beans, lentils are relatively quick to prepare. They help to manage blood sugar levels and are high in B vitamins. Lentils are loaded with folate (folic acid), essential both before and during pregnancy.

Prep time: 15 minutes
Cooking time: 25 minutes
Yield: 2 servings

1 cup dried red lentils cooked in 2 cups of water (soak for 1 hour) or 15-ounce can lentils, rinsed and drained, or chicken or turkey. (See note if you have candida.)
2 tablespoons wakame (sea vegetable)
28-ounce can of tomatoes
1 tablespoon cumin
1 teaspoon turmeric
2 tablespoons honey
½ cup raisins or chopped figs
2 cups fresh spinach

- If cooking dried lentils, add lentils and water to medium saucepan, bring to boil and simmer for 20 minutes.
- Add wakame to saucepan.
- Once lentils (or chicken or turkey if using) are cooked, add tomatoes, cumin, turmeric, honey and raisins or figs.
- Combine and cook for 5 minutes.
- Add spinach and cook, until wilted.
- Combine and serve over brown rice or brown rice pasta.

Tip

- Soaking lentils helps to fight off the gas and bloating. Make sure you throw out the soaking water before use. Rinsing the canned beans does the same thing. Adding the wakame (sea vegetable) helps to reduce gas too.

Notes

- If you have candida, omit the honey and raisins, and substitute 5 drops of stevia or to taste.
- If you have candida, avoid legumes for the first 3–4 weeks. Substitute lean protein such as 2 chicken or turkey breasts. Cut chicken or turkey into 1-inch pieces, and in a medium saucepan with 1 tablespoon of olive, sauté. until golden brown.

Quick Black Beans and Quinoa

When you are in a pinch, this is quick dinner recipe. Cook the quinoa ahead of time, and you can cook extra to mix up for a breakfast porridge with nondairy milk and maple syrup. The kale is excellent for fertility, especially for those with PCOS, as it helps to reduce inflammation.

Prep time: 25 minutes
Cooking time: 15 minutes
Yield: 4 servings

1 tablespoon olive oil
1 small onion, chopped
15-ounce can organic black beans, BPA free, drained and rinsed (Or substitute chicken or turkey. See note if you have candida.)
28-ounce can diced tomatoes
1 tablespoon basil, dried
1 tablespoon parsley, dried
1 teaspoon oregano, dried
2 cups kale, chopped
2 cups quinoa, cooked (See tip.)
sea salt and freshly ground pepper to taste

- In large saucepan, heat oil over medium heat.
- Add onion, and cook and stir, until tender.
- Add beans (or chicken or turkey if using), tomatoes, basil, parsley, oregano and quinoa.
- Simmer for 10–15 minutes.
- Add kale and cook for 2–3 minutes, until wilted.
- Serve immediately.

Tip

- To cook quinoa, rinse and drain quinoa. In medium saucepan, add 1 cup quinoa to 2 cups of water. Bring to a boil, then simmer for 15 minutes, or until water has evaporated and quinoa fluffs with a fork.

Note

- If you have candida, avoid legumes for the first 3–4 weeks. Substitute lean protein such as 2 chicken or turkey breasts. Cut chicken or turkey into 1-inch pieces, and in a medium saucepan with 1 tablespoon of olive, sauté, until golden brown.

Curry Coconut Veggies over Quinoa

This dish is hearty, heart-filled, flavourful and just plain good. There's nothing like fresh, nourishing vegetables to get the baby-makin' juices flowing. India has more than 1 billion people, so they must be doing something right! Onions, ginger and garlic are aromatic, good for your blood and cholesterol friendly. Quinoa is a complete protein that will make your body strong. This 4,000-year-old seed is a powerful aid in cell growth and repair and is an energy booster. It is packed with magnesium, iron and vitamin B6.

Prep time: 20 minutes (Depends on how fast you chop. You could use a food processor, but, sigh, it's just not the same!)
Cooking time: 25 minutes
Yield: 4 servings

1 tablespoon cold-pressed coconut oil
1 small yellow onion, finely chopped
1/2-inch piece ginger root, peeled and finely chopped
4 garlic cloves, minced
2 red potatoes, peeled and cubed (See note if you have candida.)
3 large carrots, peeled and diced (See note if you have candida.)
2–3 Roma tomatoes, peeled, seeded and diced
1 cup broccoli florets, chopped
1 cup fresh or frozen green peas (See note if you have candida.)
6 button mushrooms, sliced (See note if you have candida.)
1½ tablespoons curry powder
1 cup coconut cream or coconut milk
2 teaspoons Himalayan sea salt (optional)
1 cup quinoa, rinsed
2 cups water

- In a pot, bring quinoa and water to a boil. Reduce heat to low, cover pot with a lid and simmer for 15 minutes.
- In a large skillet, sauté onion in coconut oil over medium heat. When onions are translucent, stir in ginger and garlic.
- Cook for 5 minutes, stirring occasionally.
- Add potatoes (or turnips if using), carrots, tomatoes and broccoli.
- Stir in sea salt and curry powder.
- Cook for 10 minutes, stirring occasionally.
- Add peas (or zucchini if using), mushrooms and coconut cream.
- Cover with a lid, reduce heat to low, and cook for 10 more minutes, stirring occasionally.
- Serve hot over quinoa.

Notes

- If you have Candida, omit potatoes, carrots, peas and mushrooms. Substitute turnip and zucchini.
- The coconut cream will give it a creamy texture. The coconut milk will be less creamy. If you have access to a young green coconut, open the coconut and mix ¾ of coconut water with the soft white jelly inside. Use what is available to you, and do the best that you can with what you have!

Mexican Black Bean Enchilada

Frijoles negros, or black beans, are so full of flavour. Research has shown that animal protein reduces fertility, while vegetable protein increase fertility. Beans are an excellent source of vegetable protein. Start preparing this recipe the day before so beans have enough time to soak. Soaking reduces cooking time, increases nutrient density and reduces gas. Cooking your own beans is much healthier than using the canned version, because you can avoid excess salt and chemical such as BPAs.

Prep time: 40 minutes (after cooking beans)
Cooking time: 20–25 minutes
Yield: 4 servings

2 cups black beans, soaked for 12 hours and rinsed or 19-ounce can of black beans, organic, BPA free can, rinsed and drained (if pressed for time) (See note if you have candida.)
2 tablespoons olive oil
1 small onion, chopped
2 cloves garlic, minced
Fresh corn cut from 1 cob or ½ cup frozen
1 small green bell pepper, chopped
1 lime, freshly squeezed
½ teaspoon ground cumin
½ teaspoon chili powder
¼ teaspoon cayenne pepper (optional)
Himalayan sea salt to taste
1 jar of your favourite salsa (organic)
8 organic corn tortillas
1½ cups Daiya cheddar cheese (nondairy cheese)
Chopped fresh cilantro
1 avocado, peeled, seeded and sliced

- Cook beans either in a pressure cooker for 30 minutes or in a large pot for 60–90 minutes. Water should be 2 inches over the beans. Drain and set aside. Do not add salt because it can increase the cooking time. (Do not cook beans if using canned beans.)
- Preheat oven to 350° F.
- In a medium saucepan, sauté olive oil, onions, corn, garlic and bell pepper, until tender.
- Add beans (or chicken or turkey if using), cumin, lime, chili powder, cayenne and sea salt.
- Simmer for 2–3 minutes.
- In a 9-x-13 inch baking dish, pour enough salsa to lightly cover the bottom.
- Warm up your tortillas, one by one in a skillet, so they don't break when you bend them.
- Add about 2 heaping tablespoons of the filling to each tortilla, sprinkle with Daiya cheese, wrap and place seam side down in the baking dish. Repeat for each of the tortillas.
- Top with salsa and more Daiya cheese. Bake 20–25 minutes, until sauce is bubbling and tortillas look slightly golden.
- Sprinkle with fresh cilantro, and serve with freshly sliced avocado.

Notes

- Omit the Daiya cheese if you are omitting soy from your diet.
- If you have candida, avoid legumes for the first 3–4 weeks. Substitute lean protein such as 1 package (1 pound, or .45 kilogram) ground chicken or turkey. In a large saucepan, brown the turkey or chicken.

Moroccan Goddess Sweet Potatoes

Sweet potatoes are excellent for fertility. They contain 700% of the RDA of vitamin A, which is great for your cervical health. Beta-carotene regulates your menstrual cycle. Potassium helps reduce your feelings of stress. And much, much more. Here's a very simple recipe for getting these nutrients into your body. Be sure to wash all of your vegetables thoroughly with salt water or vegetable wash. Rinse thoroughly with water.

Prep time: 15–20 minutes
Cooking time: 35 minutes
Yield: 4 servings

1½ pounds sweet potatoes, peeled and sliced (See note if you have candida.)
4 cloves of garlic, sliced
1 red bell pepper, sliced in 4–6 pieces
1 green bell pepper, sliced in 4–6 pieces
1 small red onion, sliced
½ cup fresh flat leaf parsley, chopped
½ cup fresh cilantro, chopped
¼ cup cold-pressed extra virgin olive oil
1 tablespoon lemon juice
2 teaspoons paprika
1 teaspoon cumin
½ teaspoon Himalayan sea salt
½ teaspoon freshly ground pepper

- Preheat oven to 350° F.
- In a large bowl, mix all ingredients together.
- Pour into a lightly oiled baking dish.
- Bake for 35 minutes, or until vegetables are tender and lightly browned.

- Stir vegetables halfway through baking.
- Serve with brown basmati rice, cooked greens and garden salad.

Note

- If you have candida, substitute turnips for sweet potatoes.

Caribbean Rice and Peas

Red beans are full of fibre, protein and folate. Research suggests eating up to 3 cups of cooked beans per week. For pregnancy health, it is best to eat foods as fresh and natural as possible. I encourage cooking your own beans to reduce exposure to BPA, salt and chemicals from the canned beans, which can inhibit successful conception. I suggest cooking 2 cups of dry beans at a time, using 1 cooked cup for this recipe and freezing the rest for chili, soup and other bean recipes. Why? Because the cooking process for beans can be long. Make sure your beans are not old, or they will take forever to cook.

Prep time: 15–20 minutes
Cooking time: 25 minutes
Yield: 4 servings

2 cups red kidney beans, picked, rinsed and drained or 19-ounce BPA-free can organic kidney beans, rinsed, drained (if you are pressed for time) (See note if you have candida.)
¼ cup coconut oil
2 garlic cloves, minced
½ medium red onion, diced
2 cups uncooked long grain brown rice, rinsed
1 sprig fresh thyme
1½ cups coconut milk
2 bay leaves
Himalayan sea salt to taste
3 cups vegetable broth or water
1 teaspoon non-GMO yeast-free vegetable bouillon
1 whole Scotch bonnet pepper, chopped (optional) (See tip.)
1 teaspoon paprika

- Soak red beans for 8 to 10 hours the night before. Drain. (Omit this step and next 3 steps if you are using canned beans.) To make life easier, cook red beans in a pressure cooker or slow cooker.

- Cover beans until water is at least 2 inches higher than beans.
- Cook in pressure cooker for 1–1½ hours or slow cooker for 6 hours.
- In a skillet, heat coconut oil on medium-high heat. Sauté onions, garlic, thyme and pepper for 1–2 minutes.
- Stir in rice and beans (or chicken or turkey if using), and cook for 2 minutes.
- Add remaining ingredients, and stir.
- Bring to a boil, then simmer for 20 to 25 minutes, stirring periodically to prevent sticking and burning.
- Discard bay leaves and serve.

Tip

- Cut Scotch bonnet pepper using a knife and fork, begin careful not to get the pepper on your hands, as it may sting. Never rub your eyes or touch your tongue or any other sensitive part of your body for up to 1 hour after handling the pepper.
- If you have candida, avoid legumes for the first 3–4 weeks. Substitute lean protein such as 1 package (1 pound, or .45 kilogram) ground chicken or turkey. In a large saucepan, brown the turkey or chicken.

Bring on the Beans Hearty Chili
This is a filling meal and is even more delicious the next day. You can curl up with your sweetie and eat it by the fire, or enjoy it on a cool summer night too. Studies show that if you consume more plant-based foods, you increase your chances of conception. Bring on the beans, baby!

Prep time: 15 minutes
Cooking time: 30 minutes
Yield: 8 servings

1 tablespoons olive oil
1 small onion, chopped
2 large carrots, chopped
3 cloves garlic, minced
1 cup red bell pepper, chopped
2 stalks celery, chopped
1 tablespoon chili powder
1 tablespoon ground cumin
1½ teaspoons dried oregano
1½ teaspoons dried basil
28-ounce can organic diced tomatoes with liquid
19-ounce can kidney beans with liquid (See note if you have candida.)

- Heat oil in a large saucepan over medium heat.
- Sauté onions, carrots and garlic, until tender.
- Stir in red pepper and celery.
- Cook until vegetables are tender, about 6 minutes.
- Stir in tomatoes and kidney beans (or chicken or turkey).
- Add chili powder, cumin, oregano and basil.

- Bring to a boil, and reduce heat to medium.
- Cover, and simmer for 20 minutes, stirring occasionally.

Note

- If you have candida, avoid legumes for the first 3–4 weeks. Substitute lean protein such as 1 package (1 pound, or .45 kilogram) ground chicken or turkey. In a large saucepan, brown the turkey or chicken.

Veggie Kebabs with Brown Basmati Rice

Time for your daily serving of veggies. These veggies kebabs are packed with vitamin C, vitamin A and beta-carotene, which is essential for growth and development of the fetus. Start with a green salad or tomato soup to boost the veggies count and your fertility even more.

Prep time: 20 minutes
Cooking time: 15 minutes (45 minutes if rice not cooked)
Yield: 4 servings

Kabobs
1 red bell peppers, chopped into 4–6 pieces
1 green bell pepper, chopped into 4–6 pieces
12 button mushrooms, washed and scrubbed (See note if you have candida.)
12 cherry tomatoes
2 zucchini, thickly sliced, about ½ inch
1 red onion, chopped into 8 pieces
¼ cup olive oil

Dressing
½ cup Veganaise (mayonnaise substitute)
2 tablespoons Dijon mustard
1 tablespoon olive oil
sea salt and ground pepper to taste

Rice
1 cup of brown basmati rice
2 cups of filtered water

For Rice

- In a medium saucepan, combine rice and water.
- Bring to a boil, and simmer for 40–45 minutes, until water has evaporated and rice fluffs with fork.

For Kabobs

- Using wooden or metal skewers, assemble vegetables on four skewers.
- Brush vegetables with olive oil.
- Grill or broil for 15 minutes, turning after approximately 7 minutes.

For Dressing

- Combine Veganaise, Dijon mustard, olive oil and salt and pepper. Set aside.
- Serve kabobs on bed of basmati rice with dressing for dipping.

Note

- If you have candida, omit mushrooms.

DESSERTS AND SNACKS

Raw Energy Bars

There's a pot of gold at the end of this rainbow. (Although you may have to wait about 9 months to get it.) This bar is so nutrient dense, you and your baby will have boundless energy. Oatmeal has cholesterol-lowering fibre. Raisins contain iron and vitamin B6. Almonds are full of calcium for strong bones. Sunflower seeds are anti-inflammatory and good for your heart. Cacao helps fight depression and is high in antioxidant flavonoids, sulfur and magnesium. Pistachios are rich in copper, vitamin E and good cholesterol. And the list goes on.

Prep time: 30 minutes
Yield: 4 servings

¼ cup gluten-free oatmeal
¼ cup almonds
¼ cup pistachios
¼ cup sunflower seeds
¼ cup maple syrup
7 dates, chopped
2 tablespoons coconut oil
2 tablespoons cacao powder
¼ cup golden raisins
¼ cup cranberries or cherries, dried

- Put all ingredients, except raisins and cranberries or cherries, in the food processor or high-speed blender.
- Chop for about 30 seconds.
- Pour mixture into a bowl, and mix in raisins and cranberries or cherries.

- In a rectangular dish, spread batter evenly to ½ inch thick.
- Slice into bar shapes and place dish into the freezer for 15 minutes to hold bars together.
- Remove and eat as many as you like.
- Store remainder in the refrigerator for up to 1 week. (But they probably won't last that long.)

Notes

- If you have candida, do not consume.
- Try one of our other amazing desserts such as Strawberry Cashew Parfait.
- If you have PCOS, substitute maple syrup with 5–10 drops of stevia to taste.

Groovy Oatmeal Balls

These cookies are great for a treat or to pop in your mouth when you are on the run. Oatmeal lowers cholesterol, and research has found when cholesterol levels were lowered, healthy egg production and fertility increased.

Prep time: 10 minutes
Refrigerate: 30 minutes
Yield: 24 balls

2 cups small-flake, gluten-free oatmeal
½ cup of raisins
½ cup raw sunflower seeds
½ cup unsweetened coconut
¼ cup maple syrup
¼ cup brown rice syrup
½ cup almond butter

- Mix ingredients in medium bowl.
- Using teaspoon measurement, roll into balls.
- Place on cookie sheet lined with parchment paper.
- Refrigerate for 30 minute.
- Store in airtight container in refrigerator.

Notes

- If you have candida, omit the raisins.
- If you have PCOS and/or candida, substitute the maple syrup and brown rice syrup with 5–10 drops of stevia to taste.

Tip

- Ensure you use small flake, gluten-free oatmeal or the mixture will not form into balls
- If you only have large flake gluten-free oatmeal you can press mixture into a 9x9 baking pan. Refrigerate for 30 minutes. Cut evenly into squares.

Real Simple Chocolate Brownies

If you have a sweet tooth and need a quick (and baby-friendly) chocolate fix, then this recipe is for you. No sugar. No baking. No wheat gluten. No problem. For a little fun, give a taste to your partner with his eyes closed. He may never know these are raw. Raw and living foods maintain age-reversing enzymes and heat-sensitive vitamins and phytonutrients that are destroyed when cooked above 105° F. Nutrients from raw foods are also better absorbed by your body, so you receive the most energy that your meal has to offer. The ingredients in this recipe contain protein, natural sugars and natural stress releasers.

Prep time: 15–20 minutes
Yield: 4 servings

1 cup almond butter
2½ cups Medjool dates, pitted
½ cup cocao powder
¼ cup maple syrup

- Blend all ingredients in a food processor.
- Press evenly into a rectangular baking pan, about ½ inch thick.
- Cut into squares.
- Store in the refrigerator.
- For a divinely decadent dessert, serve with nondairy ice cream.

Note

- If you have candida or PCOS, do not consume. Try the Chocolate Chip Ice Cream or Strawberry Cashew Parfait instead.

Tip

- Ensure your Medjool dates are soft (you should almost be able to mash them with your fingers). Avoid the hard dry ones.

Strawberry Cashew Parfait
This is a crowd favourite. My family gobbles down this dessert. The fact that it is dairy free and processed sugar free and still pleases even the most finicky palate is fabulous. Strawberries are full of vitamin C, which is essential for the formation of collagen. Collagen keeps the protective membrane around the baby strong.

Prep time: 10 minutes
Yield: 4 servings

14-ounce can Thai coconut milk (Refrigerate for 24 hours,)
½ teaspoon cinnamon
2 tablespoons maple syrup for coconut milk and 2 tablespoons for cashew mixture
½ cup cashews, crushed
2 cups organic strawberries, washed and sliced

- Remove can of coconut milk from refrigerator, and turn can upside down. Open can and remove the liquid on top of the thick coconut milk (Reserve and refrigerate the coconut liquid for a smoothie.)
- In a medium bowl mix coconut for 1–2 minutes with handheld mixer, until it becomes thick and is combined.
- Add cinnamon and 2 tablespoons maple syrup, and mix for additional 30 seconds.
- In a small bowl combine cashews and remaining maple syrup.
- Place 1 tablespoon of cashew mixture on bottom of 4 bowls. Add a layer of strawberries, coconut whipped cream, another layer of cashew mixture,

strawberries and finish off with coconut whipped cream.

- Serve immediately.

Notes

- If you have PCOS and/or candida, omit the cashews.
- If you have PCOS and/or candida, substitute maple syrup with 2–3 drops of stevia in coconut mixture.

Baked Apples

These remind me of my childhood. Baked apples were often a Sunday night treat. Apples are loaded with fibre. They help keep you full longer and boost your immune system.

Prep time: 15 minutes
Cooking time: 35–45 minutes
Yield: 6 servings

6 apples (Granny Smith, pink lady or your favourite), washed and cored
½ cup raisins or currants
½ cup chopped walnuts or pecans
1 teaspoon ground cinnamon
3 tablespoons maple syrup

- Preheat oven 350° F.
- In a small bowl, mix together the raisins, walnuts or pecans, cinnamon and maple syrup.
- Place the apples in a baking dish, and stuff the core with raisin mixture.
- Bake 35–45 minutes, until apples are soft
- Serve immediately. Spoon some of the pan juices over the apples.

Notes

- If you have candida, omit the nuts and raisins. Combine ½ cup of gluten-free oatmeal flakes, 2 tablespoons melted coconut oil and cinnamon. Add ½ teaspoon of powdered stevia to taste. Stuff the mixture into apple cores.
- If you have PCOS, substitute maple syrup for 5–10 drops of stevia to taste.

Apricots with Honey
In China, apricots were called "moons of the faithful" and were thought to enhance women's fertility. They are a great source of vitamin A, vitamin C, potassium and fibre, and aid in digestion and constipation.

Prep time: 15 minutes
Cooking time: 25 minutes
Yield: 1½ cups

10–12 small, fresh, ripe apricots
2 tablespoons honey
2 teaspoons cinnamon
1 teaspoon ginger, ground

- Preheat oven to 350° F.
- Slice apricots, and place face up in baking dish.
- Evenly drizzle the honey over each apricot, filling the hollow of each half.
- Sprinkle cinnamon and ginger over the apricots.
- Bake for 15 minutes.
- Flip (be careful not to splash yourself with the hot syrup).
- Bake for another 5–10 minutes, until apricots are soft to the touch and slightly wrinkled.
- Let cool, and transfer to a covered container.

Notes

- They will keep up to 1 week in the refrigerator.
- If you have candida, do not consume. If you have PCOS, add 1 drop of stevia to apricots, or simply sprinkle with cinnamon and ginger.
- Reference: http://www.webmd.com/food-recipes/features/8-healthy-facts-about-apricots

Chocolate Chip Nondairy Ice Cream

Ahhhh. Ice cream with high-quality sugar. Feel the chocolate chips joyously dancing on your tongue! This recipe is quick, creamy and delicious. Eat as much of this healthy homemade treat as you like. Dairy contains lots of nasties (growth hormones, pesticides and viruses) that your body does not need right now. Coconut milk has lots of good healthy fats that your body will love. The blackstrap molasses has significant amounts of iron, calcium, potassium and B vitamins.

Prep time: 15 minutes plus 4–6 hours freeze time
Yield: 2 servings

2 ripe, medium-sized avocados, peeled and seeded
3 medium limes, juiced and zest (grated peeling)
1½ cup coconut milk
½ cup cacao powder
½ cup maple syrup
1 tablespoon blackstrap molasses
¼ cup nondairy chocolate (enjoy Life brand) or carob chips

- Blend all ingredients in blender, except chocolate chips.
- Pour mixture into a pan.
- Stir in chocolate chips.
- Freeze for 4–6 hours. Cover or lid is optional.
- Serve with pickles. Just kidding!

Notes

- This ice cream can be eaten alone, but it will go great with your chocolate brownies.

- There is approximately 100 milligrams of caffeine in this recipe.
- If you have PCOS and/or candida, substitute maple syrup for 5–10 drops of stevia to taste, and substitute chocolate chips for carob chips.

Banana Ice Cream with Walnuts

I love this ice cream on a warm summer day or even when I want a quick "sweet" treat. When your bananas start to ripen, peel and slice, and store in the refrigerator to make this quick treat, or pop them in your smoothies. Bananas are great for boosting sperm quality. Grab a bowl and indulge.

Prep time: 35 minutes
Yield: 2 servings

2 bananas, sliced
1 cup unsweetened almond milk or coconut milk
1 tablespoon maple syrup
2 tablespoons walnuts, chopped

- Line cookie sheet with parchment paper and lay sliced bananas on cookie sheet. Place in freezer for 30 minutes.
- Remove bananas from freezer, and place into high-speed blender.
- Add almond milk or coconut milk.
- Blend until ingredients are fully combined.
- In a small bowl, combine maple syrup and walnuts.
- Sprinkle maple syrup and walnut mixture on ice cream.
- Serve immediately.

Notes

- If you have PCOS, substitute 3–4 drops of liquid stevia, or try without, as may be sweet from banana. Add more to obtain desired sweetness.
- Do not consume if you have candida.

Fabulous Fig Yogurt

This is a quick but decadent treat. Since the time of the ancient Greeks, figs have been thought to enhance fertility. Figs are a good source of calcium and iron. Iron is important for healthy eggs and ovulation.

Prep time: 5 minutes
Soaking time: 30–60 minutes
Yield: 2 servings

6 dried figs, organic and sulphite free
1 teaspoon cinnamon
1 teaspoon vanilla
1 cup unsweetened almond milk

- Soak figs for 30–60 minutes.
- Discard soaking water.
- Combine figs, cinnamon and almond milk in high-speed blender.
- Serve and enjoy.

Notes

- Substitute 1 cup of berries for the figs if you have candida. Do not soak berries. Combine berries, cinnamon, vanilla and ½ cup of almond milk in a high-speed blender.

Va Va Voom Vanilla Pudding

According to the Aztecs, avocados are considered the ultimate fertility food. They have high vitamin E content and help with sperm motility. What are you waiting for? Time to fire up the blender.

Prep time: 5 minutes
Yield: 2 servings

1 avocado, ripe, pitted and peeled
1/3 cup unsweetened almond milk or hemp milk
2 tablespoons maple syrup
½ teaspoon cinnamon
½ teaspoon nutmeg
1 teaspoon pure gluten-free vanilla extract

- Combine ingredients in high-speed blender, and blend, until smooth.

Notes

- The pudding will be green but still delicious or you can add 1 Tbsp of cocao powder to make a chocolate pudding.
- Make sure your avocados are ripe.
- If you have PCOS, substitute maple syrup for 2–3 drops of stevia to taste.

Olive and Sundried Tomato Flax Crackers

Flax seeds have wonderful fibre to help keep your eliminatory system open and clean to meet the demands you place upon your body. They also contain omega-3 fatty acids, which are excellent for a healthy heart. Add the B-complex vitamins from the nutritional yeast for your brain and nervous system, and you have an amazingly healthy snack. These flax seed crackers are great with salads and nondairy cheese. This is a great recipe to double so you can always have some on hand.

Prep time: 20 minutes
Cooking time: 20–30 minutes
Yield: 4 servings

2 cups golden flax seeds, ground
¼ cup sun-dried tomatoes (not oil packed), chopped
¼ cup Kalamata olives, sliced
1 heaping tablespoon nutritional yeast
About 1 cup filtered water

- Preheat oven to 400° F.
- In a large bowl, mix all ingredients, except water.
- Slowly stir in water until a dough forms. You may need a little more or a little less water.
- Press dough evenly (about ¼ inch thick) into an oiled baking pan.
- Use a spatula instead of a knife to score dough into rectangles.

- Bake 20–30 minutes, until the edges are golden brown.
- Allow to cool before serving.

Note

- If you have candida, omit nutritional yeast. The recipe will still be tasty without it.

Sexy Savory Cashews
This is a quick and healthy protein-packed snack to have on hand when the munchies attack. Cashews contain zinc, magnesium and copper, which help both men and women in the fertility process. Zinc boosts semen and testosterone levels in men. Magnesium and copper help strengthen your bones and keep your elimination system clean. All 3 nutrients are great for your skin and overall pregnancy health. Soaking cashews helps to remove enzyme inhibitors, making them more easily digestible.

Prep time: 10 minutes
Drying time: 4 hours
Yield: 4 servings

2 cups raw cashews, soaked 8 hours, rinsed and drained
2 tablespoons maple syrup
½ teaspoon garlic powder
½ teaspoon paprika
¼ teaspoon cumin
A dash of sea salt

- Mix garlic, paprika and cumin a large plastic ziplock bag.
- In a bowl, mix cashews and maple syrup.
- Add cashews to the ziplock bag, seal it and shake to coat with spices.
- Remove cashews, and either dry cashews in a dehydrator at 105° F, or place in an oven on the lowest setting (200° F) for 4 hours.
- Remove and enjoy.

Notes

- If you have candida, substitute cashews for pumpkin or sunflower seeds.
- If you have PCOS and/or candida, substitute maple syrup for 2–3 drops of stevia to taste.

Traveling Trail Mix
It's always a good idea to keep a few snacks with you in case you get hungry. It takes a little bit of preparation, but it prevents that dip in blood sugar that can cause you to grab the quickest and not usually the healthiest option. The options for this trail mix are endless.

Prep time: 5 minutes
Yield: ½ cup

¼ cup almonds, whole, skin on
¼ cup macadamia nuts
1–2 tablespoons raisins

- Mix together.
- Take with you when you are on the go.
- Store in airtight glass container.

Notes

- If you have candida, you can use pumpkin seeds or sunflower seeds and omit the raisins and nuts.

Tip

- Other options include chopped or whole walnuts, cashews, Brazil nuts, or pecans, and chopped or whole currants, dates, figs or prunes.

QUICK MEAL IDEAS

Salad
Try your favourite leafy lettuce with various sliced, diced or grated veggies. The possible combinations are endless. I love adding grated carrots and sliced tomatoes and cucumbers.

- Fresh herbs are a wonderful option to mix in, as they are packed full of flavour (basil, oregano, parsley, cilantro).
- Experiment with adding diverse forms of protein to your salads such as nuts, seeds and beans. Pumpkin and/or sesame seeds are a good choice (the black sesame seeds have loads of calcium). Walnuts add some good crunch. A can of black beans or chickpeas is fast and easy when you are in a pinch.
- Pick up a light and healthy dressing at your local health food store, or mix up something easy, like lemon juice, black pepper and olive oil. Another option is walnut or flax oil mixed with unpasteurized apple cider vinegar (2 tablespoons of oil to 1 teaspoon vinegar).
- Sea vegetables pack some healthy protein and yummy flavour. Dulse flakes sprinkle nicely and give the salad a delicious taste of the sea.

Soup
In large saucepan, saute one chopped onion with minced garlic. Chose a few of the following ingredients such as beans, lentils, potatoes, carrots, kale, spinach, canned tomatoes or any leftover vegetables. Add vegetable stock to cover ingredients. Season with bay leaves, salt and herbs such as cumin or basil and oregano. Simmer for 15–20 minutes. Serve with toasted gluten-free bread and Earth Balance nondairy butter.

Pasta
Cook up your favourite gluten-free noodles, then add a sauce such as tomato, pesto or herbs and oil such as olive oil, walnut oil or avocado oil. Add in chickpeas, lentils or nuts. Toss in some steamed kale, spinach or Swiss chard.

Sandwiches
Start with gluten-free bread. Add a spread such as mashed avocado, hummus, a store-bought dip, nondairy butter such as (Earth Balance) or vegan mayo (Veganaise). Next add cucumber, lettuce, sprouts, avocado or tomato. Include a favourite condiment such as sauerkraut or salsa, and add salt and pepper to taste.

Stir Fry
Stir fries are fast and tasty. Add 1 tablespoon oil, sauté 1 small chopped onion and 2 cloves of minced garlic for 3-4 minutes until onion is translucent. Add some cubed tempeh for protein. Throw in your favourite fresh vegetables, . Sauté until tender. Add ½ cup of water for a sauce. For flavour add 2 tablespoons of tamari to taste. Add greens such as spinach and kale near the end, as they don't take very long to cook. Serve on brown rice, quinoa or pasta.

Rice Bowl/Noodle Bowl

Fill a bowl with cooked brown rice or noodles. Add steamed greens (kale, spinach), toasted seeds and avocado slices. Top with oil such as walnut or avocado and unpasteurized apple cider vinegar or tamari.

Note: brown rice takes 40 minutes to cook, and rice noodles take about 10 minutes. Quinoa is another good grain to try and takes only 15–20 minutes.

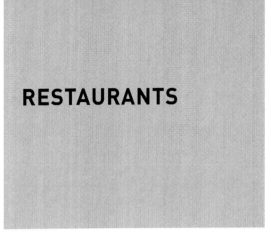

RESTAURANTS

Basically, when I go into a restaurant, I don't look at the menu and ask the server what they recommend. It is more difficult to eat vegan and gluten-free in most restaurants, but vegetarian (fish, rice and veggies) is a lot easier. Most servers are very accommodating when you specify your dietary requirements. Yes, you become "high maintenance," but when you eat food that heals you instead of harms you, you feel a whole lot better, and that's a good thing!

Vegan Restaurants
http://www.happycow.net/north_america/
Gluten-free restaurants:
http://www.theceliacscene.com/gluten-free-sitemap.html

Email me at sarah.clark@sesacoaching.ca if you want recommendations for my favourites.

ADDITIONAL RECIPE WEBSITES

Not all of these sites are vegan, but many offer many gluten-free options.

http://ohsheglows.com/
https://www.drfuhrman.com/library/recipes.aspx
www.vegweb.com
www.vegkitchen.com
www.thehealthyhappywife.blogspot.ca
www.elanaspantry.com
www.thekindlife.com
www.rickiheller.com
http://againstallgrain.com/recipe-index/
http://kblog.lunchboxbunch.com/

INDEX